ACLS Essentials
Basics and More

ACLS Essentials
Basics and More

Kim McKenna
RN, BSN, CEN, EMT-P

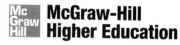

McGraw-Hill
Higher Education

Boston   Burr Ridge, IL   Dubuque, IA   New York   San Francisco   St. Louis
Bangkok   Bogotá   Caracas   Kuala Lumpur   Lisbon   London   Madrid   Mexico City
Milan   Montreal   New Delhi   Santiago   Seoul   Singapore   Sydney   Taipei   Toronto

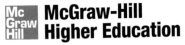

McGraw-Hill
Higher Education

ACLS Essentials–Basics and More

Published by McGraw-Hill, a business unit of The McGraw-Hill Companies, Inc., 1221 Avenue of the Americas, New York, NY 10020. Copyright © 2008 by The McGraw-Hill Companies, Inc. All rights reserved. No part of this publication may be reproduced or distributed in any form or by any means, or stored in a database or retrieval system, without the prior written consent of The McGraw-Hill Companies, Inc., including, but not limited to, in any network or other electronic storage or transmission, or broadcast for distance learning.

Some ancillaries, including electronic and print components, may not be available to customers outside the United States.

Medicine is an ever-changing science. As new research and clinical experience broaden our knowledge, changes in treatment are required. The authors and the publisher of this work have checked with sources believed to be reliable in their efforts to provide information that is complete and generally in accord with the standards accepted at the time of publication. However, in view of the possibility of human error or changes in medical sciences, neither the authors nor the publisher nor any other party who has been involved in the preparation or publication of this work warrants that the information contained herein is in every respect accurate or complete, and they are not responsible for any errors or omissions or for the results obtained from use of such information. Readers are encouraged to confirm the information contained herein with other resources, including drug-related information.

Every effort has been made to secure permissions for borrowed material. We wish to thank the associations and individuals who provided permission for us to borrow their materials.

This book is printed on acid-free paper.

1 2 3 4 5 6 7 8 9 0 DOC/DOC 0 9 8 7

ISBN 978–0–07–299932–7
MHID 0–07–299932–2

Publisher: *David T. Culverwell*
Senior Sponsoring Editor: *Claire Merrick*
Developmental Editor: *Michelle L. Zeal*
Outside Developmental Services: *Julie Scardiglia*
Senior Marketing Manager: *Lisa Nicks*
Senior Project Manager: *Kay J. Brimeyer*
Senior Production Supervisor: *Kara Kudronowicz*
Designer: *Laurie B. Janssen*
Cover Designer: *Ron Bissell*
(USE) Cover Image: *©Masterfile Royalty Free, Illustration ©The McGraw-Hill Companies, Inc.*
Compositor: *Carlisle Publishing Services*
Typeface: *10/12 Myriad*
Printer: *R. R. Donnelley Crawfordsville, IN*

All photos are © The McGraw-Hill Companies, Inc./Rick Brady, photographer.

Library of Congress Cataloging-in-Publication Data

McKenna, Kim.
    ACLS essentials–basics and more / Kim McKenna.
       p. cm.
    ISBN 978–0–07–299932-7 — ISBN 0–07–299932–2
       1. Cardiovascular emergencies. 2. Cardiac resuscitation. I. Title.

RC675.M355 2008
616.1'025–dc22

2006047062

www.mhhe.com

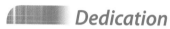 *Dedication*

For my parents

Anne and John Tubman

I am always challenged to model your love for family and friends, your dedication to your community, and your willingness to give your all—whether at work or at play.

Kim McKenna

About the Author

Kim McKenna serves as the Director of Education for St. Charles County Ambulance District in metropolitan St. Louis, Missouri. For the previous six years, Kim was the Chief Medical Officer for a fire-based EMS program. She has been a registered nurse for more than 30 years, with clinical experience in emergency and critical care nursing and, for the past 20 years, in prehospital and emergency education. Kim is an active member of the National Association of EMS Educators and is the editor of their scholarly publication, *Domain3*.

Brief Contents

Contents

3 Respiratory Distress and Arrest   22

4 Public Access Defibrillation   44

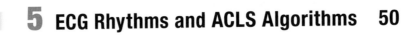

5 ECG Rhythms and ACLS Algorithms 50

6 Acute Coronary Syndromes 94

10 Special Resuscitation Situations   164

ACLS Algorithms

Chapter 8

Chapter 10

Foreword

As stakeholders in healthcare professions, our commitment to providing quality patient care gives us a diversity of responsibilities. As healthcare practitioners, whether novices or experts, providers or educators, we are challenged to protect the communities in which we serve by integrating existing medicine and new knowledge fostered by research.

In this text, *ACLS Essentials—Basics and More,* Kim McKenna effectively and eloquently compliments the research-based 2005 American Heart Association guidelines in a concise and systematic format.

All advanced practitioners will find this text an essential resource for successful completion of ACLS training. The Basic and Advanced Life Support concepts and skills emphasized throughout the text will provide the paramedic, registered nurse, and physician with the foundation to challenge ACLS with confidence.

This text not only focuses on the established standard of care, but identifies alternatives for further action beyond the algorithm. The incorporation of mnemonics promotes easy retention of information. The tables, which provide an explanation of the signs and symptoms and common causes of cardiac dysrhythmias, enhance the interpretation of simple and complex ECG rhythms.

The inclusion of an anatomy and physiology review provides a relevant foundation for chapters that discuss presentations of acute coronary syndromes (ACS) and stroke. Chapter 4 emphasizes the importance of the Public Access Defibrillation programs and the application of Basic Life Support knowledge and skills outside the healthcare environment. Chapter 5 includes a logical and fundamental approach to 12-lead ECG interpretation. The emphasis on cardiac anatomy, and how it relates to the ECG changes, provides an easy method of recognizing the inclusion and exclusion criteria for effective management. The clinical features of stroke provided in Chapter 7 identify typical and atypical conditions that mimic stroke etiology.

The experienced practitioner and educator will appreciate the in-depth discussion of classic and nonclassic presentations of complicated coronary syndromes and stroke. Discussion of variances in electrolyte disturbances, maternal resuscitation, complicated respiratory etiologies, rapid sequence intubation, hypothermia, and termination of resuscitation efforts enhance the ACLS foundation of knowledge.

Special features like *Testing Tips* and *The Bottom Line* in each chapter effectively summarize the key concepts and critical actions necessary for better understanding of ACLS concepts.

Appendix A provides a quick-reference ACLS Medications Table. The *Notes* section within the table provides rationales and critical actions for "thinking outside the box" for ACLS medication administration. The alphabetical summary of common ACLS abbreviations found in Appendix B provides a reference for rapid identification and understanding of ACLS terminology.

This patient-care-focused text provides a dynamic tool to easily review the in-depth knowledge needed for mastery of ACLS concepts. Entry-level and experienced practitioners alike will find this text helpful in identifying critical actions for safe practice for patients experiencing ischemic stroke, acute coronary syndromes, and lethal arrhythmias. *ACLS Essentials—Basics and More* will help build practitioners' confidence in providing quality patient care and demonstrating competency in the knowledge and skills required for successful completion of ACLS training.

Linda M. Abrahamson, BA, RN, EMT-P
EMS Education Coordinator, Silver Cross Hospital
Adjunct Faculty, Joliet Junior College
Joliet, Illinois
Past President, National Association of EMS Educators (NAEMSE)

Preface

ACLS Essentials—Basics and More, and the materials that accompany it, are designed for you to review, refresh and enhance the knowledge you need to care for adult patients who have emergency cardiovascular conditions. You may use the materials for individual study, but they are best supplemented with an Advanced Cardiac Life Support class, where you will have the opportunity to practice the skills necessary to provide effective emergency cardiac care.

ACLS Essentials—Basics and More is divided into 10 chapters, supplemented with two appendixes. Each chapter provides essential information related to a specific aspect of emergency cardiac care in a concise, step-by-step format. Chapters 1 through 7 review core material that is essential for the first 10 minutes of cardiovascular emergency care. The illustrations enhance critical content to promote understanding of the material. Chapters 8 through 10 outline considerations for ongoing care and address the special considerations involved in caring for patients who have conditions that result from complex causes.

The two appendixes enhance the chapters and provide you with rapid reference materials in an easy-to-access format. Appendix A contains information about drugs that are commonly used in emergency cardiac care. The drugs are listed alphabetically by generic and common trade names. Drug actions, uses, adult dose, common side effects, and notes that reflect important considerations for emergency administration are included. The design allows you to find essential information at a quick glance. Information that is italicized refers to special care considerations that an experienced ACLS provider would need to know. Appendix B provides a ready reference of abbreviations, listed alphabetically so you can quickly find their meaning while reading the textbook or during clinical practice.

Supplementary content provided on the DVD that accompanies this text includes a review of many skills discussed in this book. Watch the skills on the DVD to help you learn or review each skill. The flashcards on the DVD will help you prepare for testing if you are studying for an Advanced Cardiac Life Support program. In addition, the accompanying CD provides 251 self-test multiple-choice questions with an answer key and brief rationale for each answer. Use the practice questions to assess your knowledge related to Advanced Cardiac Life Support.

I hope this text improves your knowledge of emergency cardiac care and that it will help you feel confident when you are studying for ACLS training. The ultimate goal of this book is to better prepare you to provide effective care to patients who have life-threatening emergency cardiac conditions.

Enjoy!

Kim McKenna, RN, BSN, CEN, EMT-P
Director of Education
St. Charles County Ambulance District
St. Louis, Missouri

Supplements

Student DVD

- Essential skills for ACLS packaged in the back of the text
- Includes Digital Flashcards

Student CD

- 251-question self-test multiple-choice exam with answer key and rationales

Acknowledgments

The preparation of this text and the accompanying support materials was a collaboration of some great emergency care and publishing professionals. Thanks to all who helped:

- Thanks to Jeanne Shepard for writing the CD questions, to Angie Elliott for writing the DVD flashcards, and to Jon Politis for input on the DVD video skills. Your assistance is greatly appreciated.
- The quality and completeness of this book were enhanced by the professional evaluations of the emergency care professionals who reviewed this project. My thanks to them for their helpful feedback.
- Delve Productions, led by Steve Kidd, John Czajkowski, and Alex Menendez, have crafted careful, straightforward skills videos that will be of great benefit to healthcare professionals, especially those who do not provide emergency care on a daily basis.
- To my husband, Don, and my children, Ginny, Becky, Maggie, and Grant, thanks for pitching in and putting up (again) with the interruptions to our lives while I completed this text.
- To Janet Schulte, "the Empress of all things American Heart" at St. Charles County Ambulance District, I appreciate your responding so quickly 24/7, in true EMS fashion, to my questions as I prepared this manuscript.
- To all of my coworkers and students, past and present, who challenge me every day to question why we do things so we can be our best—you have taught me so much.
- Thanks to Kay Brimeyer and Laurie Janssen of McGraw-Hill for all their hard and excellent work in the production and design of this text.

- Wendy Nelson provided the eagle eye in copyediting to ensure a clear, consistent text for the readers.
- The rich illustrations developed for this text by Imagineering will help the reader understand difficult content.
- Thanks to Claire Merrick for allowing me this opportunity—and for just being Claire.
- Last, and most importantly, I owe a debt of gratitude to the vision, diligence, attention to detail, and professionalism of Julie Scardiglia, developmental editor. Her ability to clearly articulate expectations, suggest improvements, provide gentle reminders, and clarify difficult concepts contributed greatly to this text.

Kim McKenna, RN, BSN, CEN, EMT-P
Director of Education
St. Charles County Ambulance District
St. Louis, Missouri

Reviewers

Linda M. Abrahamson, BA, RN, EMT-P
EMS Education Coordinator, Silver Cross Hospital
Adjunct Faculty, Joliet Junior College
Joliet, IL

Angie Elliott, RN, EMT-P
Elliott Resource Group, Inc.
Eustis, FL

Janet Fitts, RN, EMT-P, Educational Consultant
Prehospital and Emergency Medical Services
Pacific, MO

Donna Gilbert
Anne Arundel Hospital Center
Annapolis, MD

Lynn D. Kidd, RN, BSN
Apopka, FL

Gail Orum-Alexander, PharmD
Charles R. Drew University of Medicine and Science
Los Angeles, CA

David S. Pecora, PA-C, NREMT-P, RN
Chief, Physician Assistant
Dept. of Emergency Medicine, West Virginia University
Fairmont, WV

Jeanne Shepard
Mesa Fire Department
Mesa, AZ

Keith Wesley, MD, FACEP
Wisconsin State EMS Medical Director
Madison, WI

Jim Whaley, RPh
Baker College
Owosso, MI

Introduction to ACLS

1

Passing ACLS

The American Heart Association (AHA) created the Advanced Cardiac Life Support (ACLS) course so that healthcare providers can learn the clinical foundation upon which to base their management of patients who either are in cardiac arrest or are in danger of having a cardiac arrest. This management includes care of the cardiac arrest victim, the patient who presents with chest pain, the patient who has a serious condition that may lead to cardiac arrest, and the patient who has been successfully resuscitated from cardiac arrest. The recognition and treatment of ischemic stroke and the use of automated external defibrillators (AEDs) are also included. The ACLS course does not certify that you are proficient in any of the skills and techniques contained in the program; it merely certifies that you have received the educational content and have successfully demonstrated your understanding of the concepts. The true purpose of the course is to ensure that you have a firm understanding of ACLS fundamentals. In fact, the primary goal of ACLS training is for you to feel comfortable caring for a patient during the first 10 minutes of a cardiac arrest.

ACLS Testing

Successfully completing your ACLS course will require you to demonstrate a basic understanding of the initial assessment and management of the following ten skills and emergency situations:

1. Respiratory Distress
    - This includes shortness of breath and respiratory arrest.
2. Automated External Defibrillation
    - This station also offers the opportunity to reinforce your CPR skills.
3. Ventricular Fibrillation and Pulseless Ventricular Tachycardia
4. Pulseless Electrical Activity (PEA)

5. Asystole
6. Acute Coronary Syndromes (ACS)
7. Bradycardia
8. Unstable Tachycardia
9. Stable Tachycardia
10. Acute Ischemic Stroke

In addition to the skills and scenarios noted above, the experienced ACLS provider will be required to demonstrate the care and management of patients suffering from the following conditions:

- Toxic overdose
- Trauma
- Hypothermia
- Hyperthermia
- Metabolic abnormalities
- Severe asthma
- Anaphylaxis

Your knowledge will be evaluated in two ways: through a written exam and through demonstrating critical patient care skills via staged scenarios (the mega code station).

The Written Exam

For many individuals, the written exam is the easiest part of the course. However, some individuals get test anxiety and become confused by the multiple-choice questions. The point of the exam is to ensure that you understand the concepts. Read the questions carefully, and be sure to select answers that address the priorities of care in the right order: airway, breathing, circulation, and, if needed, defibrillation. If you do not achieve a passing score on the first test, an instructor will review the answers with you. You will be given time to review the material and then be reevaluated.

Critical Patient Care Scenarios (Mega Code)

Some courses include a station (or stations) where you may be randomly presented with any ACLS scenario. During the patient situation, you will be the team leader—responsible for guiding your team members through the proper assessment and care of the patient. For some students, this is the most intimidating and anxiety-producing portion of the course. The next section deals with tips for successfully completing these scenarios.

Successfully Navigating Critical Patient Care Scenarios (Mega Code)

The most important key to successfully managing a stressful situation is to first take a deep breath and remember the basics. Remember that the situation can only improve if you remain calm, cool, and collected. Use the following tips when you are being evaluated during an ACLS program or anytime you are faced with a real-life ACLS patient:

- Listen closely as the evaluator reads the scenario (or to the patient's history, if you are caring for a real patient). If necessary, make written notes to remind yourself of any unique or unusual aspects of the case.

- Start each ACLS scenario or patient encounter with the primary ABCs. Determine the patient's responsiveness. Call for help if the patient does not respond.

- Assess the patient to see if he or she is breathing, and check for a pulse.

- If there is no pulse, immediately have someone begin CPR and bring the defibrillator to the bedside.

- Take your time. Do not hurry through any stage of the scenario or any part of patient care. Examine the cardiac rhythm, as well as the patient's history, signs, and symptoms. Then make your diagnosis. This step is critical. It will set the stage for each subsequent action by determining which algorithm (treatment plan) you will use. If you fail to gather the proper information or you misinterpret your assessment findings, you will choose the wrong treatment path and you may harm your patient.

- State each rhythm you encounter out loud so that your teammates or the instructor understand which algorithm you are using. Better yet, verbally indicate to the group which algorithm you are using so there is no confusion.

- The algorithms provide a framework or pathway to follow to provide appropriate patient care for a given condition or rhythm. The algorithm will suggest the medications you will need to give. Request that they be administered at their proper time, dose, and rate.

- It is your responsibility to be familiar with the medications you are giving in every patient care situation. Along with the dose, route, and rate, you must know any contraindications to the use of the drug, understand how it may interact with other drugs the patient is taking, and know what side effects to anticipate. If you don't know, look it up! Just as you have a reference book with you during your ACLS training and testing, you should always have one handy while caring for real patients.

- Check for a pulse at the appropriate intervals.

- Remember: You are providing patient-focused care—not machine-focused care. Evaluate the success of all of your interventions based upon how the patient is responding to them (not on how the machines are responding). If the patient is conscious, how does he or she feel? Are the patient's general appearance and color improving?

- Ensure that defibrillation or cardioversion is delivered in a safe manner. Unsafe delivery of electrical therapy is a critical error in mega code.

- If there is a pulse, then there must be a blood pressure. Assess vital signs often if a pulse is present.

- Move methodically through the algorithm. Do not hurry. The most important thing you can do if you cannot remember the next step is to ensure that adequate CPR is being performed, and that the patient is being oxygenated and ventilated at the proper rate. Take this time to repeat (to yourself or out loud) the steps you have already taken, and decide which intervention to use next. If appropriate, ask your teammates for suggestions about how to proceed—this might not be an option while you're being evaluated during a class, but during real-life patient care situations it should be part of the process.

 ## Using the Algorithms

Even though you will have a reference guide with you—ideally, even in a real-life situation—there is often no time during the first few minutes of a critical emergency to pause and look things up. Memorize the algorithms so that you can provide rapid, appropriate emergency cardiac care. Doing so is also critical so that you can anticipate the logical sequence of events that should occur during the management of each scenario. The problem for many ACLS providers is that the algorithms are written in a stepwise manner that does not accurately reflect real-life cases. During an actual resuscitation, many actions take place simultaneously. You will need to take this into consideration when performing the case studies in a classroom setting. Think of the algorithms as a mental checklist of things you and your team should do or consider doing for your patient. The following list of suggestions may help you move smoothly through the algorithms:

- If the patient is in cardiac arrest, remind yourself of the following steps: "Begin effective CPR, ventilate the patient, intubate when you can, and start an IV."
- When defibrillating, always use safe techniques and state *"I'm clear, you're clear, everyone is clear!"* while simultaneously looking up and down the patient's body to ensure that no one is touching the patient. Watch the patient, not the monitor, when you activate the defibrillator.
- If the patient had a pulse and the rhythm changes, first check for a pulse, and then decide which algorithm to follow.
- If you are unsure where to begin, it is acceptable to start at the beginning of the algorithm so that you do not omit any critical steps.
- If the rhythm changes, you may start at what looks like the most appropriate point in the new algorithm. Keep in mind the actions you have already taken. For example, if the case starts out as ventricular fibrillation and you have started CPR, defibrillated and intubated the patient, and administered epinephrine, and the patient's rhythm changes to asystole, then continue with atropine and repeat epinephrine at the appropriate intervals.
- At some point—either when you have moved completely through the algorithm and the patient has failed to respond, or when you have successfully resuscitated him and feel that you have done everything to make the patient as stable as possible—stop and take a moment to review your care and decide if there is anything else to be done. When you are satisfied that you have accomplished all that can be done, inform the evaluator that you are finished. Tell the instructor what should be done next: pronounce the patient dead; or move the patient to the emergency department or intensive care unit; or transfer the patient to another facility for definitive care.

- If you resuscitate the patient and at some earlier point you administered an antiarrhythmic medication, determine if a continuous infusion of an antiarrhythmic is indicated. If no antiarrhythmic was administered and the patient was in a rhythm that would have qualified for an antiarrhythmic agent, administer one-half of the usual loading dose and institute a continuous infusion.
- Tachycardias are a common post-resuscitation rhythm and are the result of circulating adrenergic agents as well as the patient's endogenous epinephrine secretion. They rarely require treatment and therefore should only be monitored closely. Administer an antiarrhythmic agent if it is indicated.

ACLS Team Management

Providing ACLS is a team effort. Success in ACLS is greatly enhanced if you have an effective team of rescuers, each with a specific role to play. In your practice setting, the number of team members and their qualifications may vary widely. You will have to adapt your approach to patient care depending on the resources you have available at any given time in the resuscitation. Regardless of the team makeup or size, someone has to take charge. Without an effective team leader, there will be no overall coordination of care, and steps may be overlooked or inappropriate treatment may be given. While the instructor is evaluating your ability to progress appropriately through the algorithms, he or she will also be assessing your overall management of the code as a team leader. Being a team leader requires that you do the following:

- Take charge of the scene.
- Assign responsibilities to each of your team members.
- Control the actions of bystanders.

These actions allow you to maintain a position of oversight to ensure that the code progresses smoothly. It also ensures that you are aware of each action performed on your patient and that your orders are carried out safely. As a team leader, you will usually be responsible for the following:

- Interpreting cardiac rhythms
- Ordering medication administration
- Safely delivering defibrillation or cardioversion
- Assessing proper endotracheal tube placement

Assign a team member for each of the following activities:

- Performing CPR
- Maintaining the airway
- Establishing intravenous or intraosseous access and administering medications
- Recording a written, chronological list of the actions performed, the medications administered, their results, the patient's vital signs, and all rhythm interpretations
- Crowd control, if needed

As team leader, you must understand the ethics of resuscitation. In particular, you must know the role of advance directives and Do Not Resuscitate (DNR) orders. When you are the team leader, you must recognize when resuscitation should stop and when it should not be initiated at all. This requires an understanding of local protocols and practices. You may be called on to counsel family and friends of the patient; you should therefore understand the role of grief counseling.

In addition, as team leader, you must communicate effectively and respectfully with team members. You must be able to critique the code using positive communications skills. Evaluate what went well and ask the team to identify performance that could have been improved. This may require waiting some time after the code rather than discussing it immediately following the arrest, when tensions may be high and team members may not be in a receptive mood.

The team leader must also be able to recognize signs of stress in team members and must be prepared to counsel them or ensure that they receive qualified counseling following the event.

Most importantly, you must inspire confidence in the team.

ACLS Troubleshooting

At some point in your experience with ACLS, you will feel that everything is going wrong and that your actions are not producing the desired outcomes. When this occurs, it is vital that you step back, reevaluate the situation, and look for the cause of this confusion. To prevent problems or identify areas where you may encounter difficulty, perform the following actions:

- Ensure that adequate CPR is being performed. Watch for rescuer fatigue that may hinder adequate perfusion and rotate rescuers to the chest compression role every 2 minutes. Use CPR assist devices if they are available and your team is trained in their use. Minimize interruptions in CPR.
- Keep your hand on the patient's pulse at all times so that you will know immediately if the patient loses her or his pulse.
- If the patient is intubated, frequently reassess the proper placement of the endotracheal tube through auscultation and by using other measures such as end-tidal CO_2. When you move the patient, the tube might shift from the trachea into the hypopharynx or esophagus. Check for correct tube placement after each patient move.
- Ensure that the oxygen delivery device is connected to the oxygen source and that oxygen is flowing to it.
- Verify that the cardiac monitor leads are properly connected and that the defibrillation pads are making adequate contact with the patient. Make sure the cardiac monitor is in paddle mode when defibrillation pads are being used to monitor the rhythm.
- Ensure that intravenous lines are patent and have not infiltrated. If in doubt, establish another point of vascular access.

◇ ◇ ◇ **Testing Tips**

- Read your pre-course textbook materials carefully.
- Familiarize yourself with the handbook or pocket guide that you will use during ACLS—you'll need to know where to find things quickly.
- Memorize the algorithms related to arrest and peri-arrest (the period leading up to cardiac arrest or immediately after the return of spontaneous circulation).
- State your interventions aloud as you perform them so the evaluator and your team members know exactly what you are doing.
- Assign team roles early.
- Monitor team performance continually.
- Ensure that adequate CPR is performed with minimal interruptions.
- Reassess the patient and your plan of care often.

The Bottom Line

You are taking ACLS because you provide healthcare in a setting with patients at risk for cardiac arrest or other cardiac emergencies. Study the ACLS algorithms and drugs, and practice the ACLS skills. Your goal for this course should be to gain the knowledge and skills to care for a real patient who is in cardiac arrest or to prevent a patient from having a cardiac arrest. That's an important responsibility. If you study this text carefully, you will be closer to that goal.

2

ACLS Fundamentals

To successfully care for patients who need Advanced Cardiac Life Support, you must remember the fundamentals. No matter how complex the case or how hectic the scene, if you follow the essential steps of ACLS, you will know that you treated the patient appropriately, no matter the outcome. Memorize the ACLS fundamentals in this chapter and use them in every ACLS situation. While you should refer to resource materials to ensure that you administer the proper drug doses, you must understand the initial steps to follow and the appropriate drugs to use.

Chain of Survival

The patient's chance for survival increases when the following elements of emergency cardiac care are in place in your community (Figure 2-1):

- Early access
- Early CPR
- Early defibrillation
- Early advanced care

5-Step Approach to ACLS

Follow this process when you assess each ACLS patient, and you will gather the essential information and perform the initial steps you need to begin appropriate care:

1. Primary ABCD survey
2. Secondary ABCD survey
3. Oxygen, IV, monitor, fluids
4. Vital signs (temperature, blood pressure, heart rate, respiratory rate)
5. Rate, volume (tank), pump

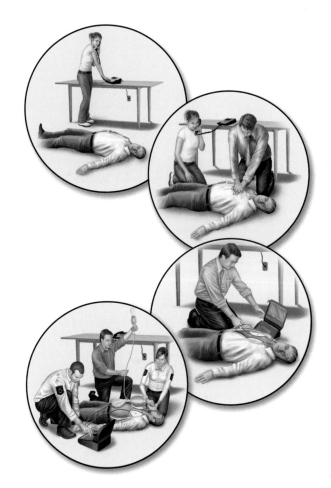

FIGURE 2-1   The Chain of Survival.

Primary ABCD Survey

Healthcare providers often focus on advanced skills and medications and overlook the basics of ACLS. You must not miss these steps if you wish to have a good patient outcome:

A

- **A**ssess responsiveness
- **A**ctivate EMS (911)
- **A**cquire defibrillator
- **A**irway (open)

B

- **B**reathing
  - Positive-pressure ventilation if not breathing

C
- **C**heck pulse
  - Chest compressions if no pulse

D
- **D**efibrillate pulseless ventricular tachycardia (VT)/ventricular fibrillation (VF)

Airway

1. Open the airway using the head tilt–chin lift maneuver.
2. If you suspect an injury to the neck, attempt to open the airway using the jaw-thrust without head-tilt maneuver first.

Breathing

1. Look, listen, and feel for breathing for up to 10 seconds.
2. If there is no breathing, give 2 breaths deep enough to make the chest rise.
3. Use a pocket mask or bag-mask to ventilate.
4. If there is a pulse, deliver rescue breathing at a rate of 1 breath every 5–6 seconds.

Circulation

1. Feel for the patient's pulse at the carotid artery for no longer than 10 seconds.
2. If there is no pulse, begin chest compressions:
   - Place two hands over the sternum, between the patient's nipples.
   - Compress 1 ½ to 2 inches deep.
   - Push hard and fast (100 times per minute).
   - Allow full chest recoil after each compression.
   - Avoid interrupting CPR.

   See Table 2-1 for the sequence of adult CPR.

TABLE 2-1 Adult CPR Sequence

Airway	Use the head tilt–chin lift maneuver.
Breathing	Assess for < 10 seconds. Give 2 breaths at 1 second each.
Circulation	Perform a pulse check for < 10 seconds.
Compressions	Give 100 per minute at a depth of 1 ½ to 2 inches.
Ratio of compressions/ ventilation	30:2 for one or two rescuers.
Compressions/ventilations (with an advanced airway)	Give 100 compressions per minute. Give 1 breath every 6–8 seconds.

Defibrillation

During ventricular fibrillation, random, rapid, electrical depolarization makes the heart quiver chaotically. This prevents organized contraction of the heart, stops effective blood flow, and causes immediate cardiac arrest. Rapid delivery of electrical defibrillation of the heart simultaneously depolarizes a critical mass of myocardial cells. This allows the normal pacemakers to resume their rhythmic, coordinated function.

You increase defibrillation success by delivering the first shock very quickly, and by ensuring that effective cardiopulmonary resuscitation is performed.

 ## Secondary ABCD Survey

Airway

- Insert the airway device when possible after initial CPR and defibrillation.

Breathing

- Confirm placement of the airway device by clinical assessment methods plus mechanical devices.
- Provide positive-pressure ventilation.
- Evaluate the effectiveness of ventilation.

Circulation

- Establish IV/IO access.
- Apply a cardiac monitor and identify the rhythm.
- Administer appropriate drugs.

Differential diagnosis

- Search for and treat the cause of the condition.

 ## Critical Tasks of Resuscitation

During a cardiac arrest, or when caring for a critically ill cardiac patient who is at risk for sudden cardiac arrest, a sequence of rapid critical interventions must be performed to enhance the patient's chance for survival. To be effective, your team must perform these tasks in a fast, safe, proper, and organized format. There is no time to "figure things out" in the middle of a patient resuscitation—you must be prepared to perform the following interventions before the crisis begins:

- Airway management
- Chest compressions
- Monitoring and defibrillation
- Vascular access and medication administration

Treatment Classifications

The American Heart Association has assigned the following treatment classifications to selected interventions throughout ACLS. These classifications are based on clinical research and expert consensus.

- **Class I:** Definitely recommended; the benefits definitely outweigh the risks
- **Class IIa:** Acceptable and useful; the benefits outweigh the risks
- **Class IIb:** Acceptable to consider; the benefits are at least as great as or possibly more than the risks of use
- **Indeterminate:** Promising, but sufficient evidence is lacking; research is ongoing
- **Class III:** May be harmful; the risk is greater than the benefit; not recommended

 # ACLS Medication Administration

IV/IO Drug Administration

Start a peripheral IV line if your patient has had a sudden cardiac arrest.

- If you are unable to establish peripheral IV access, and you have the appropriate training and supplies, you may place an intraosseous (IO) needle.
- Placing an intraosseous needle involves inserting a special needle into the marrow cavity of the bone.
- You can then administer fluids and medications as you would through an IV line.

Drug Administration During Cardiac Arrest

- During cardiac arrest, most drugs are given IVP.
- After you give the IV drug, elevate the arm and flush the tubing with 20 mL of normal saline.

Endotracheal Medications

You may administer several resuscitation drugs through the endotracheal tube (ETT). When you give drugs by the ET route, the absorption and therefore the effects are not predictable.

- Give drugs by the IV or IO route if possible.
- The dose for endotracheal administration is usually 2 to 2½ times the intravenous dose.
- Dilute the drug with 5–10 mL of sterile water or normal saline and administer it via the endotracheal tube.

The following drugs may be given by the endotracheal route:

- **N**aloxone
- **A**tropine
- **V**asopressin
- **E**pinephrine
- **L**idocaine

◇ ◇ ◇ **Testing Tips**

- Think of "NAVEL" to remember the drugs that you may give via the ET tube:

  Naloxone

  Atropine

  Vasopressin

  Epinephrine

  Lidocaine

Defibrillation

When you defibrillate a patient, electric current is delivered through the chest to the heart. The flow of current through the heart causes depolarization of the myocardial cells. Ideally, a normal underlying heart rhythm will then resume. This energy charge is delivered from the defibrillator capacitor through either metal paddles or adhesive patches (hands-free).

Defibrillation Success

Successful defibrillation depends upon the following:

- Time to the first shock
  - Survival declines 7–10% each minute from collapse to the first shock if no CPR is performed.
  - Deliver the first shock as quickly as possible for a witnessed arrest.
- Effective cardiopulmonary resuscitation
  - Survival decreases 3–4% each minute from arrest to the first shock if CPR is performed.[1]
  - Perform CPR for 2 minutes before defibrillation if the arrest is unwitnessed.
- An effective level of energy delivery
  - The amount of energy needed to defibrillate varies according to the defibrillation waveform.

---

[1] American Heart Association, "AHA Guidelines for Cardiopulmonary Resuscitation and Emergency Cardiovascular Care," *Circulation* 112, suppl. 1 (2005).

Monophasic Versus Biphasic Defibrillators

There are several types of current waveforms that can be used to defibrillate. Research is under way to determine how the waveform affects a defibrillator's ability to successfully convert ventricular tachycardia and fibrillation. The monophasic defibrillator sends the energy from one electrode to the other in one direction. It does this without taking into consideration the size of the patient or the body's resistance to conducting the energy (impedance).

Biphasic defibrillators alternate the direction (polarity) of the electrical energy as it is delivered. The biphasic defibrillator also measures the impedance (resistance to the flow of electric current) across the patient's chest and compensates so that more energy is delivered to the heart itself. These properties allow biphasic defibrillators to successfully defibrillate at lower energy levels than monophasic defibrillators.

It is important to know what type of defibrillator waveform you are using to treat your patient. Select the energy levels recommended by the manufacturer of the specific device you are using. If the defibrillator is biphasic but you don't know the manufacturer's energy recommendation, defibrillate at 200 J.

Assessing the Initial ECG Rhythm in Cardiac Arrest

When your patient is in cardiac arrest, you must rapidly determine his or her ECG rhythm. If you are already monitoring the patient, you can quickly glance at the monitor to interpret the rhythm. However, if your unmonitored patient suddenly and unexpectedly arrests, you can waste precious time connecting the limb ECG monitoring leads. In these situations, use the quick-look method to determine the patient's ECG rhythm.

Quick-Look Method

If your patient is unresponsive and pulseless, you may perform a "quick look" to see the rhythm if the ECG monitor is not already connected.

1. After you turn the monitor on, choose "Paddles" on the lead selector.
2. Attach the adhesive defibrillation patches or place the paddles with the conductive medium on the chest as you would to defibrillate.
3. Look at the monitor screen to see the rhythm.
4. Prepare to charge and defibrillate if indicated.
5. Attach the limb ECG electrodes as soon as possible and change the lead selector to the lead you wish to monitor.

◇ ◇ ◇ **Testing Tips**

- Hold the paddles firmly in contact with the chest if you are using the "quick-look" mode to assess the rhythm. If you lift the paddles, the rhythm will appear to be asystole.

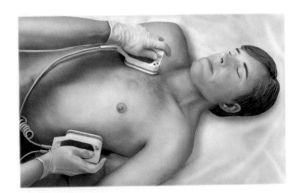

FIGURE 2-2   Defibrillation using manual paddles.

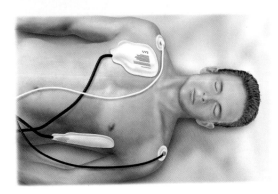

FIGURE 2-3   Defibrillation using hands-free patches.

Defibrillation Technique

The technique for defibrillation will vary depending on whether you are using manual paddles or self-adhesive (hands-free) defibrillation patches. The two most common methods are the use of manual paddles (Figure 2-2) and hands-free defibrillation (Figure 2-3).

Defibrillation Using Manual Paddles

1. Turn on the power to the monitor/defibrillator.
2. Determine that the rhythm is VF or VT.
3. Verify that the patient has no pulse.
4. Apply conduction gel to the paddles or pre-gelled conduction pads to the patient's chest.
5. Select the appropriate energy level.
6. Place the paddles on the patient's chest.
   - Anterior–anterior (sternum–apex): Place the sternum paddle below the right clavicle. Place the apex paddle in the left midaxillary line to the left of the nipple.
7. Apply firm pressure.

8. Press the charge button while reassessing the rhythm.
9. Call *"I'm clear, you're clear, everyone is clear!"* while looking head to toe to ensure that no one is touching the patient
10. Resume CPR.
11. Check the rhythm after 2 cycles of CPR and defibrillate again if indicated.

Hands-Free Defibrillation

1. Turn on the power of the monitor/defibrillator.
2. Determine that the rhythm is VF or VT.
3. Verify that the patient has no pulse.
4. Place the adhesive defibrillation pads on the patient's chest in the anterior–anterior (sternum–apex) position or in the anterior–posterior position.
   - Anterior–posterior patch position: Place one patch over the apex of the heart (the center should be over the point of maximal impulse). Place the second patch on the patient's back, directly opposite the first and to the left of the thoracic spine.
5. Connect the adhesive pads to the defibrillation cable and ensure that the cable is connected to the monitor/defibrillator.
6. Select the appropriate energy level.
7. Press the charge button while reassessing the rhythm.
8. Call *"I'm clear, you're clear, everyone is clear!"* while looking head to toe to ensure that no one is touching the patient.
9. Press the shock button.
10. Resume CPR.
11. Check the rhythm after 2 cycles of CPR and defibrillate again if indicated.

Defibrillation Indications and Energy Levels

The indications and energy levels for the defibrillation of adults are provided in Table 2-2.

TABLE 2-2 Defibrillation—Adult

Indications	Pulseless ventricular tachycardia Ventricular fibrillation Hemodynamically unstable polymorphic ventricular tachycardia
Energy levels	Monophasic defibrillator: 360 J Biphasic defibrillator: 120–200 J (based on the manufacturer's recommendations) ■ Biphasic rectilinear waveform: 120 J ■ Biphasic truncated waveform: 150–200 J ■ If unknown biphasic defibrillator: 200 J Deliver subsequent doses at the same or higher energy level

◇ ◇ ◇ **Testing Tips**

- First, *do no harm!* You must be sure that neither you nor any of your teammates are touching the patient when you defibrillate or cardiovert.
- Don't stop CPR while the defibrillator pads are applied or during the time the defibrillator is charging.

Synchronized Cardioversion

Synchronized cardioversion is used to cardiovert patients with a pulse who have a rapid atrial or ventricular rhythm that is causing hemodynamic compromise. When you deliver synchronized cardioversion, the shock is timed to avoid the relative refractory period of the cardiac cycle. This timing reduces the risk that the shock could cause ventricular fibrillation. To use the synchronizer mode, follow these steps:

1. Turn on the monitor and ensure that there is a tall R wave in lead II.
2. Administer sedation if time and the patient's condition permit.
3. Press the synchronizer button.
4. Watch to see that the QRS complex has been marked (indicated by a small line or triangle on the R wave).
5. Apply the defibrillation paddles or self-adhesive pads as for defibrillation.
6. Select the appropriate energy level.
7. Call *"I'm clear, you're clear, everyone is clear!"* while looking head to toe to ensure that no one is touching the patient.
8. Depress the shock button(s) and hold until the shock is delivered.
9. Reassess the patient and the rhythm.

Indications and Energy Levels

The ECG rhythms and their associated energy levels indicated for adult synchronized cardioversion are listed in Table 2-3.

TABLE 2-3   Synchronized Cardioversion—Adult

ECG Rhythm	Energy Levels*
Paroxysmal supraventricular tachycardia (PSVT)	50–100–200–300–360 J
Atrial flutter	50–100–200–300–360 J
Atrial fibrillation	100–200–300–360 J
Monomorphic VT with pulse	100–200–300–360 J

*or equivalent biphasic shocks

Testing Tips

- If you press the button(s) to deliver a synchronized cardioversion and no shock is delivered, check to be sure that:
    - You held the button(s) down until the shock was delivered.
    - The R wave is being marked by the machine in the lead you are monitoring.
    - The patient is still in an organized rhythm that is suitable for this treatment.

Transcutaneous Pacing

A transcutaneous pacer is used to stabilize the bradycardic patient until a transvenous pacemaker is inserted.

Indications

Transcutaneous pacing is used in patients with hemodynamically significant bradycardia that is:

- Unresponsive to atropine
- Mobitz type II second-degree or third-degree AV block with a wide QRS
- Severely symptomatic
- Associated with a ventricular escape rhythm that is symptomatic

Transcutaneous pacing is used infrequently to treat polymorphic tachycardic rhythms that are unresponsive to other therapies.

- Be prepared to provide transcutaneous pacing (with the pacer ready and, in some cases, the pacer pads applied) for a patient who is having a myocardial infarction if you observe any of the following:
    - Type II second-degree heart block
    - Third-degree AV block
    - New or unknown intraventricular conduction blocks (right or left bundle branch block or bifascicular block)

Pacing is not indicated for patients with the following conditions:

- Severe hypothermia (pacing may cause ventricular fibrillation)
- Asystolic cardiac arrest

Pacemaker Technique

1. Before you attempt pacing, ensure that the patient is monitored using limb leads.
2. Explain the procedure to the patient.
3. Apply self-adhesive defibrillation/pacing pads to the patient's chest.
    - Use either the anterior–anterior position or the anterior–posterior position.

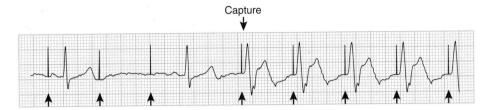

FIGURE 2-4 Transcutaneous pacing. When electrical capture occurs, the narrow pacer spike is followed by a wide QRS complex.

4. Start with a rate of about 70–80 bpm.
5. Slowly increase the current (mA) until capture occurs (a wide QRS complex and a wide T wave after each pacer spike) (Figure 2-4).
   - Increase the current setting by 2 mA after initial capture is seen.
6. Assess the femoral pulse to confirm mechanical capture after electrical capture is seen.
7. Reassess the patient's signs, symptoms, and vital signs.
8. If the patient is conscious, administer analgesics or sedate with a benzodiazepine, if appropriate.

◇ ◇ ◇ **Testing Tips**

- If you see ECG capture, verify that there is mechanical capture by checking for a pulse.
- If you use the anterior–posterior patch position for transcutaneous pacing, assess the patient's vital signs on the right side—there will be less interference from muscle contractions on that side.

Adjuncts to Improve Circulation

There are several commercial devices that may be used during cardiac arrest in an attempt to improve circulation. Three of these devices are the impedance threshold device, the band or vest CPR device, and invasive perfusion devices.

Impedance Threshold Device

The impedance threshold device (ITD) has a Class IIa AHA recommendation when it is used on intubated patients in cardiac arrest. The ITD contains a valve that has been demonstrated to improve systolic blood pressure, cerebral blood flow, and survival to the ED. Attach the ITD between the endotracheal tube and the bag-valve device or ventilator. Remove the device if the patient regains spontaneous circulation and breathing.

Band and Vest CPR Devices

Vest CPR devices have a band that encircles the patient's chest and is attached to a backboard. When you activate the device, it constricts the patient's chest at regular intervals. It delivers consistent chest compressions and minimizes the need to interrupt CPR. The AHA has assigned the load-distributing band CPR device a Class IIb recommendation.

Extracorporeal CPR Techniques

The AHA recommends invasive perfusion devices as a Class IIb intervention for patients who have an inhospital cardiac arrest if they can be initiated quickly and if the cause of arrest is reversible or treatable with a heart transplant or coronary artery bypass graft.

The Bottom Line

To successfully resuscitate the ACLS patient, you will need an organized, systematic approach. Each step in your care, from basic airway techniques through advanced electrical therapies, should be performed at the right time and in the right manner. Only then will your patient have the best chance for recovery.

3

Respiratory Distress and Arrest

At some point in your career, you will be required to assess and manage a patient suffering from respiratory distress or respiratory arrest with a pulse. You will also need to demonstrate that you can perform these skills in your ACLS course. To provide proper care during this scenario, you'll need to accomplish the following:

1. Open the patient's airway. Determine if it is clear.
   - Listen for airway sounds that indicate an obstruction (snoring, gurgling, etc.).
   - Look for matter in the airway that may obstruct air flow (blood, vomit, etc.).
2. Assess the patient to see if she or he is breathing: Look, listen, and feel.
3. Establish whether the patient is breathing effectively: Are the rate and depth of respirations adequate?
   - Oxygen saturation levels provide you with useful information, but they may not indicate adequate ventilation. Pulse oximetry does not measure carbon dioxide levels that rise during respiratory failure. End-tidal CO_2 monitoring devices can help you assess ventilation.
4. Determine if the airway is maintainable.
   - The level of consciousness is the best indicator of the patient's ability to maintain a patent airway.
5. Apply supplemental oxygen if the patient is hypoxic. If the airway is not maintainable, insert an appropriate airway device. Assist ventilation if the patient is not breathing adequately using the appropriate device for the situation. You may need to:
   - Apply a nasal cannula or mask for a conscious patient who has adequate, spontaneous breathing.
   - Perform manual airway maneuvers.
   - Deliver bag-mask ventilation using the appropriate rate and tidal volume.
   - Insert an airway adjunct if the patient requires assisted ventilation.
   - Insert, or assist with the insertion of, an alternative advanced airway device (within your scope of practice).
   - Insert, or assist with the insertion of, an endotracheal tube (within your scope of practice).
6. Monitor the patient's response to your interventions. Make adjustments if needed based on the patient's condition.

Indicators of Respiratory Distress

It is important to recognize signs of respiratory distress early. If you detect and treat breathing difficulty early, you can prevent respiratory failure.

Indications of respiratory distress include the following:

- Respiratory rate > 25 or < 8
- Oxygen saturation < 90%
- End-tidal CO_2 level > 40
- Decreased level of consciousness or restlessness (hypoxia and/or metabolic and respiratory acidosis)
- Audible wheezing
- Increased work of breathing (retractions or other accessory muscle use)
- Skin color changes (cyanosis, pallor)

Oxygen Delivery Devices

Common oxygen delivery devices, along with their approximate flow rate and the percentage of oxygen they supply, can be found in Table 3-1.

TABLE 3-1 Oxygen Delivery Devices

Device	Flow Rate	Oxygen %
Nasal cannula	1–6 L/min	24–44%
Simple face mask	6–10 L/min	40–60%
Partial rebreather mask	6–10 L/min	35–60%
Nonrebreather mask	10–15 L/min	60–100%
Bag-mask	15 L/min	up to 100%

Manual Airway Maneuvers

Open the airway using manual maneuvers first. Manual airway maneuvers include the head tilt–chin lift and jaw thrust without head tilt.

Head Tilt–Chin Lift

Use the head tilt–chin lift to open the airway of a patient with no suspected neck or head trauma:

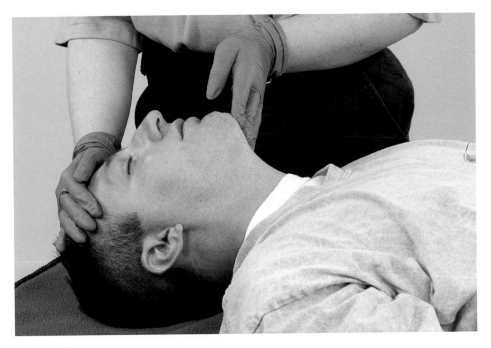

FIGURE 3-1   Head tilt–chin lift maneuver.

1. Place one hand on the patient's forehead and the other on the bony prominence under the chin.
2. Lift the chin while tilting the head back (Figure 3-1).

Jaw Thrust Without Head Tilt

If you suspect neck trauma, use the jaw thrust without head tilt to open a patient's airway:

1. Maintain the head in a neutral position.
2. Place your hands on either side of the patient's face.
3. Grasp behind the angles of the patient's jaw and pull the mandible forward (Figure 3-2).

If you can not open the airway using the jaw thrust, use the head tilt–chin lift.

 ## Basic Airway and Ventilation Devices

After you open the airway with a manual maneuver, insert the appropriate basic airway device. These devices include the oropharyngeal airway (OPA), nasopharyngeal airway (NPA). If it is necessary to assist the patient's ventilation use a pocket mask or bag mask.

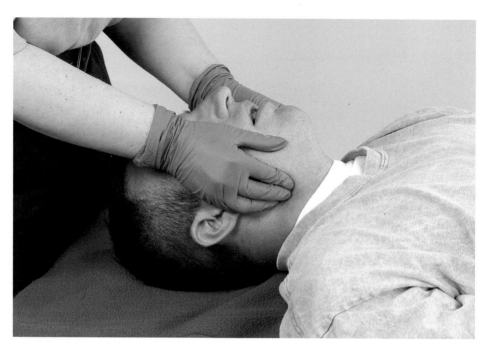

FIGURE 3-2 Jaw-thrust maneuver.

Oropharyngeal Airway (OPA)

Oropharyngeal airways may be used in unconscious patients who do not have a gag reflex.

OPA Insertion

To insert an OPA, follow these steps (Figure 3-3):

1. Open the patient's airway using a manual maneuver.
2. Select the correct-size OPA by measuring the device from the corner of the mouth to the angle of the jaw.
3. Invert the OPA so that its tip points to the roof of the mouth, and insert it into the patient's mouth.
4. When the tip reaches the junction of the hard and soft palate, rotate it 180 degrees and advance the OPA until the flange is at the teeth.
5. Reassess the patient for adequate breathing.

Alternate insertion method:

1. Depress the tongue with a tongue blade.
2. Insert the OPA along the angle of the tongue until the flange is at the teeth.
3. Reassess the patient for adequate breathing.

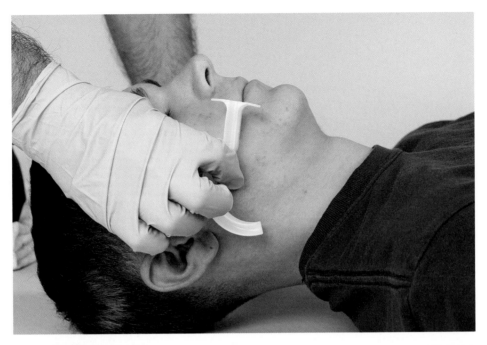

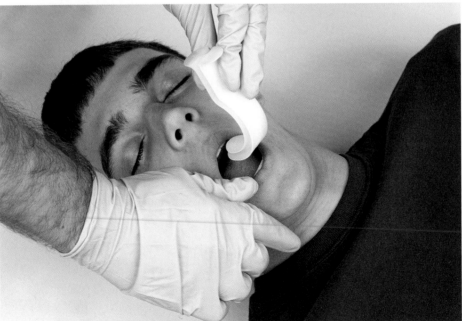

FIGURE 3-3 Inserting an oropharyngeal airway.

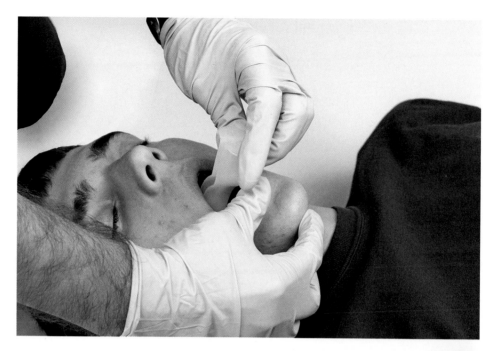

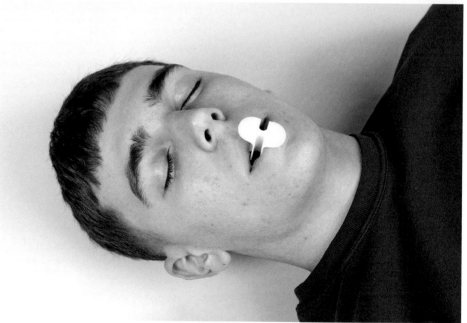

FIGURE 3-3 *(continued)*

Nasopharyngeal Airway (NPA)

Nasopharyngeal airways are used to help maintain a patent airway when the patient is semiconscious with a gag reflex (e.g., stroke, drug overdose).

NPA Insertion

To insert an NPA, follow these steps:

1. Select a size of NPA that will fit in the patient's nare.
2. Lubricate the NPA with a water-soluble gel.
3. Insert it gently into the largest nare, with the bevel toward the septum until the flange rests against the nare (Figure 3-4).
4. Reassess the patient for adequate breathing.

◆ ◆ ◆ **Testing Tips**

- Start with basic airway maneuvers and progress to advanced.
- Each time you insert any airway device, reassess the patient's breathing.

Pocket Mask

You can use a pocket mask with a one-way valve to deliver ventilation when a bag-mask ventilation device is not available. The one-way valve will prevent patient vomitus from entering your mouth. Some pocket masks have an oxygen inlet that allows supplementary oxygen delivery. One rescuer can maintain an effective mask seal and ventilate adequately using this device.

Pocket Mask Ventilation

To ventilate using a pocket mask, follow these steps (Figure 3-5):

1. Position yourself at the patient's head.
2. Use a manual airway technique to position the patient's head.
3. Set the pocket mask on the patient's face, with the point over the bridge of the nose and the flat end of the mask between the patient's lower lip and chin.
4. Position your thumbs over either side of the mask, beside the patient's nose and pointing toward the eyes.
5. Place your pointer (index) fingers on either side of the bottom of the mask.
6. Place your other three fingers on each hand under the patient's mandible.
7. Lift the patient's jaw while firmly pressing down on the mask so that it seals against the patient's face.
8. Deliver a breath over 1 second (to make the chest rise):
   - Give 1 breath every 5–6 seconds if the patient has a pulse.
   - Give 2 breaths after every 30 chest compressions if the patient is pulseless.

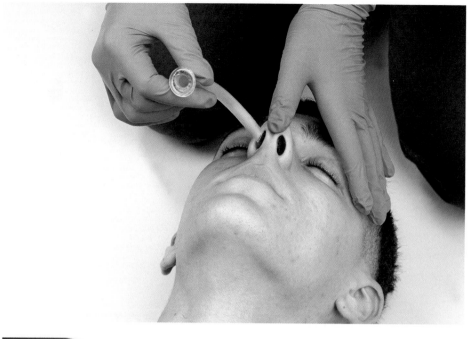

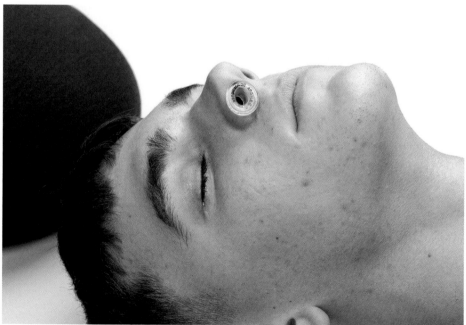

FIGURE 3-4 Inserting a nasopharyngeal airway.

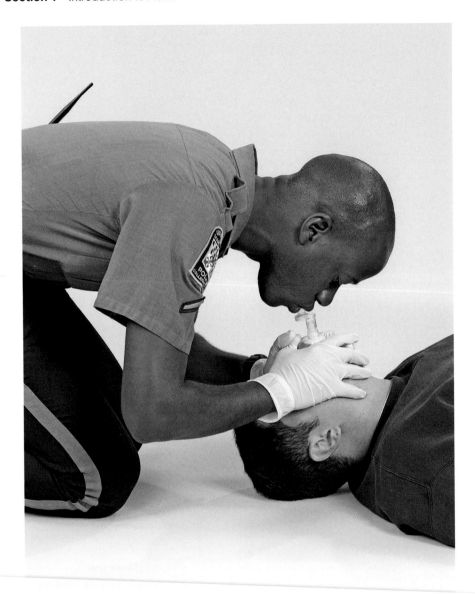

FIGURE 3-5   Ventilation using a pocket mask.

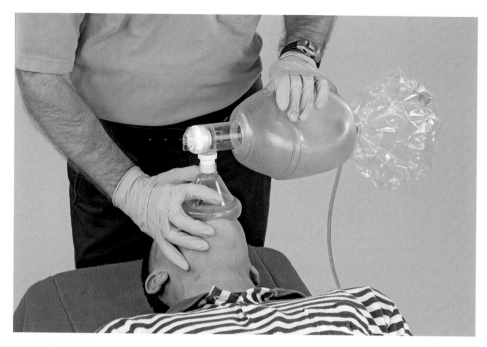

FIGURE 3-6   One-person bag-mask ventilation.

Bag-Mask

Use the bag-mask device to ventilate patients who have inadequate breathing or are apneic. Connect the bag-mask device to supplemental oxygen as soon as possible. If you have trouble maintaining a good mask seal, you may not be able to deliver adequate ventilation. In that case, have another rescuer use two hands to maintain a good mask seal while you squeeze the bag to ventilate at the proper rate.

Bag-Mask Ventilation—One Rescuer

To ventilate using a bag mask with the one-rescuer method, follow these steps (Figure 3-6):

1. Set the pocket mask on the patient's face with the point over the bridge of the nose, and the flat end of the mask between the lower lip and chin.
2. Position your thumb and pointer finger around one side of the mask in a "C" shape.
3. Place your other three fingers of the same hand under the patient's jaw to form an "E" shape.
4. To get a good mask seal, press down firmly on the mask with the fingers that are forming the "C" as you lift the jaw with the fingers that form an "E."
5. Squeeze the bag with the other hand to deliver 6–7 mL/kg volume with each breath (until you see adequate chest rise).

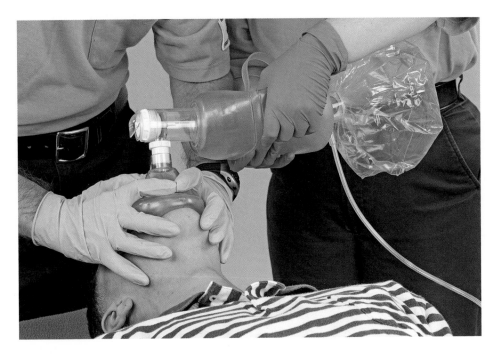

FIGURE 3-7   Two-person bag-mask ventilation.

6. For a patient with a pulse, deliver 1 breath every 5–6 seconds. During CPR, deliver 2 breaths after every 30 compressions.
7. Connect oxygen 15 L/min to the bag-mask device as soon as possible.

Bag-Mask Ventilation—Two Rescuers

To ventilate using a bag mask with the two-rescuers method, follow these steps (Figure 3-7):

1. Position yourself at the top of the patient's head.
2. Set the pocket mask on the patient's face with the point over the bridge of the nose, and the flat end of the mask between the patient's lower lip and chin.
3. Place your thumbs over either side of the mask, beside the patient's nose and pointing toward the eyes.
4. Position your pointer fingers on either side of the bottom of the mask.
5. Place your other three fingers on each hand under the patient's jaw.
6. Lift the patient's jaw while firmly pressing down on the mask so that it seals against the patient's face.
7. The second rescuer will ventilate at 6–7 mL/kg (until there is adequate chest rise).
8. For a patient with a pulse, deliver 1 breath every 5–6 seconds. During CPR, deliver 2 breaths after every 30 compressions.
9. Connect oxygen to the bag-mask device as soon as possible.

◇ ◇ ◇   **Testing Tips**

- Monitor your rate of ventilation—people tend to ventilate too quickly.
- Allow 1 second to deliver the breath.
- The correct volume for ventilation is just enough to make the chest rise.

Endotracheal Tube (ETT)

Insert an endotracheal tube if you need to protect the patient's airway and allow delivery of effective ventilation. You may also use it as an alternate route for administration of naloxone, atropine, vasopressin, epinephrine, or lidocaine. Consider intubation when:

- You are unable to ventilate the patient adequately with a bag-mask.
- The patient has no protective airway reflexes.
- You anticipate the need for prolonged ventilation.

Insertion of the Endotracheal Tube

To insert an endotracheal tube, use these steps:

1. Pre-oxygenate and, if necessary, ventilate the patient until it is time to intubate.
2. Gather your equipment and check it to ensure that it is working properly.
3. Position the patient in the sniffing position.
   - Head elevated 10 cm with flexion of the lower neck and extension of the head at the atlantooccipital joint.
4. Grasp the laryngoscope handle in your left hand.
5. Open the patient's mouth with your right hand.
6. Insert the lighted laryngoscope blade into the right side of the patient's mouth.
7. Use the blade to sweep the patient's tongue to the left.
8. Advance the laryngoscope blade to the proper position and lift:
   - Curved blade: Into the vallecula
   - Straight blade: Lift the epiglottis
9. Visualize the vocal cords.
10. Advance the endotracheal tube until the cuff passes through the vocal cords.
11. Remove the laryngoscope blade.
12. Inflate the pilot balloon with 6–10 mL of air.
13. Note the depth (cm marking) of the tube at the teeth.
14. While holding the tube, ventilate using a bag-valve device and confirm tube placement.
15. Secure the tube.
16. Reconfirm tube placement after each patient movement or change in condition.

17. Continue ventilation at the proper rate and volume.
- For a patient with a pulse: 10–12 breaths per minute
- For a pulseless patient: 8–10 breaths per minute without pausing CPR

◇ ◇ ◇ **Testing Tips**

- If endotracheal intubation is not within your scope of practice, you will not be evaluated on this skill. You will be expected to know how to assist with intubation and how to confirm proper ET tube placement.

Confirming Endotracheal Tube Placement

Use both clinical assessment and confirmation devices to ensure that the endotracheal tube is placed properly in the trachea. Reconfirm placement each time the patient is moved. This is a responsibility of all ACLS providers. A misplaced endotracheal tube can result in death. It is *critical* to do both clinical and device confirmation of tube placement—not to pass ACLS, but to ensure that you don't harm your patient!

Clinical Assessment Methods

To perform the clinical methods to assess tracheal tube placement, you'll need to observe the chest and auscultate the chest and epigastric area using a stethoscope while ventilations are delivered:

- Directly visualize the endotracheal tube passing between the vocal cords.
- Observe for adequate chest rise and fall with ventilation.
- Auscultate breath sounds bilaterally in the anterior chest and in the midaxillary region.
- Listen for the absence of epigastric sounds with ventilation.
- Feel for compliance of the bag-valve device.

Table 3-2 lists breaths sounds that confirm proper endotracheal tube placement.

Mechanical Confirmation Devices

No single method to detect tracheal tube placement is completely reliable, so you must use at least one device immediately after intubation to confirm that the endotracheal tube is located in the trachea. Ideally, you should perform continuous device monitoring of tube placement so you will know if the tube becomes dislodged during patient care or movement.

Confirmation devices include:

- Pulse oximetry
- End-tidal CO_2 measurement

TABLE 3-2 **Breath Sound Confirmation of Endotracheal Tube Placement**

Auscultation of Breath Sounds	Interpretation	Action Needed
Present and equal over both lungs	Suggests proper placement in trachea	No action is needed.
Present over right lung; absent over left lung	Suggests right mainstem intubation	Deflate the cuff and retract the tube several millimeters until bilateral breath sounds are audible.
No breath sounds audible over right or left lung	Suggests the tube is not in the trachea	Deflate the cuff and remove the tube. Ventilate and reintubate the patient.

- Esophageal detector device
  - Use before delivery of the first breath after ET intubation.
- Chest X-ray

Figure 3-8 provides examples of endotracheal tube confirmation devices. Table 3-3 provides information about confirming endotracheal tube placement using the esophageal detector device and the end-tidal CO_2 reading.

◇ ◇ ◇ Testing Tips

- With colorimetric end-tidal CO_2 detectors, remember:
  - Yellow = YES! (good tube)
  - Tan = Trouble (check the tube)
  - Purple = Problem (pull the tube)
- If the Glasgow coma score is "less than 8, intubate!"
- Reconfirm tube placement often.
- If the patient's condition and oxygen saturation begin to drop, use the "DOPE" mnemonic to find the cause:
  - **D**isplacement—Did the endotracheal tube become displaced from the trachea?
  - **O**bstruction—Is the tube obstructed with fluids that need to be suctioned?
  - **P**neumothorax—Did the patient develop a pneumothorax?
  - **E**quipment—Is there an equipment problem? Is the oxygen disconnected, is the tubing kinked, or is there a problem with the ventilator?

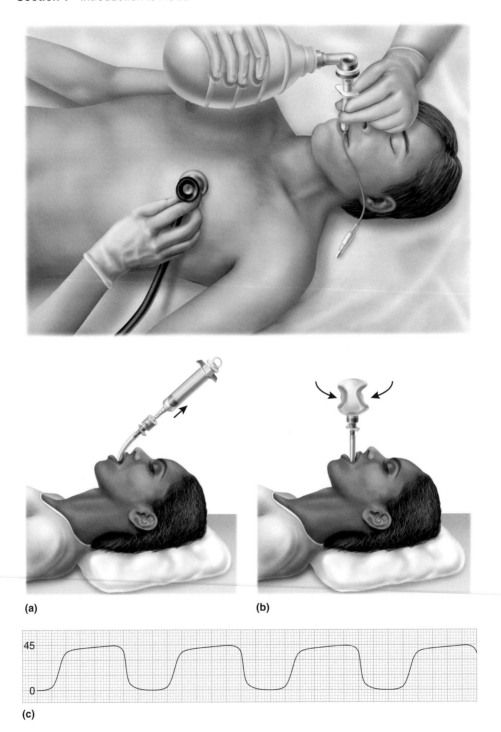

(a)

(b)

(c)

FIGURE 3-8 Endotracheal tube confirmation methods. (a) Auscultation of lungs, (b) confirmation using a bulb esophageal detector device, and (c) confirmation using capnography.

TABLE 3-3 Interpreting the Esophageal Detector Device and the End-Tidal CO_2 Reading when Confirming Tube Placement

Device	Reading	Interpretation
Colorimetric end-tidal CO_2	No color change after 6 ventilations are delivered.	Suggests the tube is not positioned in the trachea; may not be accurate in cardiac arrest.
	Color change with each ventilation.	CO_2 is present; tracheal placement is likely—continue ventilation.
Capnography	Plateau-shaped waveform is present; end-tidal CO_2 level is detected and displayed.	Tracheal placement is highly probable—continue ventilation.
	No end-tidal CO_2 waveform with each ventilation; no end-tidal CO_2 level is detected.	Strong possibility that tube is in esophagus—remove the endotracheal tube.
Esophageal detector device bulb	Bulb refills immediately after it is compressed.	Suggests tracheal placement—continue ventilation.
	Bulb remains collapsed.	Esophageal placement is likely—remove the endotracheal tube.
Esophageal detector device syringe	Plunger can be withdrawn easily.	Suggests tracheal placement—continue ventilation.
	Plunger is difficult to withdraw.	Suggests esophageal placement—remove the endotracheal tube.

 # Alternative Advanced Airways

Alternative advanced airways include the esophageal-tracheal Combitube and laryngeal mask airway. These airways provide an alternative airway to emergency providers who are not trained in, or whose scope of practice does not include, endotracheal intubation. These airways can also be used to establish an airway in situations where direct visualization of the vocal cords is impossible because of edema, blood, tissue damage, or anatomic distortion.

Esophageal-Tracheal Combitube (ETC)

The esophageal-tracheal Combitube (ETC, or Combitube) is a dual-lumen airway device that you insert blindly without visualizing the vocal cords (Figure 3-9). It is the most frequently used, nonvisualized airway device in the prehospital setting. It offers an alternative airway if you are unable to perform endotracheal intubation.

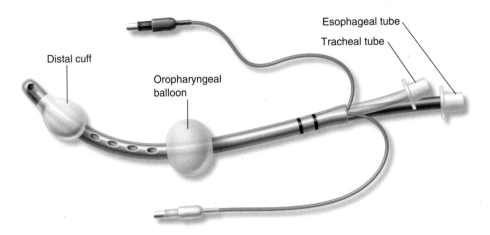

FIGURE 3-9   Esophageal-Tracheal Combitube (Combitube).

The Combitube is a double-lumen tube with an esophageal obturator lumen and a tracheal lumen. The esophageal obturator lumen is blocked at the distal end and has perforations at the level of the pharynx. The tracheal lumen is open at both ends. A large oropharyngeal balloon seals the mouth and nose. The distal cuff seals either the esophagus or the trachea, depending on placement. The Combitube is inserted blindly into the oropharynx until the printed ring marks on the tube lie between the front teeth. The oropharyngeal balloon is then inflated. After you insert the Combitube, you must assess the patient to determine through which lumen to ventilate the patient. The lumen used depends on whether the distal tip of the Combitube is resting in the esophagus or in the trachea.

Combitube Insertion

To insert a Combitube, use the following steps :

1. Select the appropriate size tube:
   - 37 Fr for patients 4–5 feet tall
   - 41 Fr for patients taller than 5 feet
2. Test the balloons to ensure there are no leaks. Lubricate the distal tip of the Combitube.
3. Place the patient's head in a neutral position.
4. Insert the Combitube blindly. Pass it down the back of the patient's mouth until the teeth line up between the two black rings on the Combitube.
5. Inflate the proximal pharyngeal balloon (the blue lumen or #1 tube) with 100 cc of air and the distal esophageal balloon (the white/clear lumen or #2 tube) with 15 cc of air.

Follow these steps to select the correct lumen to ventilate when using the Combitube:

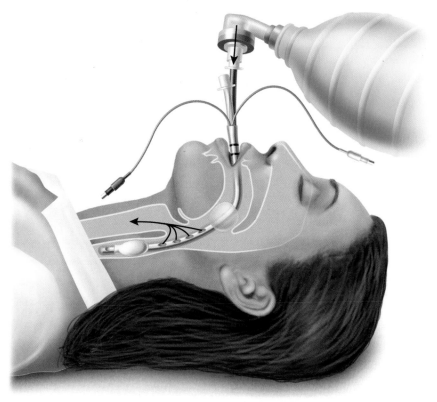

FIGURE 3-10 Combitube, esophageal placement.

1. First, ventilate the patient through the blue lumen (tube #1). If the Combitube is in the esophagus, as it most frequently is, air will pass through the proximal holes and into the trachea (Figure 3-10).
   - Check for breath sounds in the high axillary areas bilaterally and over the epigastrium.
   - You should hear breath sounds in the chest, *not* bubbling over the stomach.
   - If you hear bubbling over the stomach, then move to step 2.
2. Ventilate the patient through the white or clear lumen (tube #2) (Figure 3-11). If the Combitube is in the trachea, you will hear breath sounds in the chest; you will *not* hear bubbling over the stomach.
3. If in doubt, attempt ventilation through each lumen while auscultating the lungs and the epigastrium.

Laryngeal Mask Airway (LMA)

The laryngeal mask airway may be used in the following situations: (1) in routine and emergency anesthetic procedures, (2) in known or unexpected difficult airways, and (3) to establish an airway during resuscitation in the unconscious patient with absent

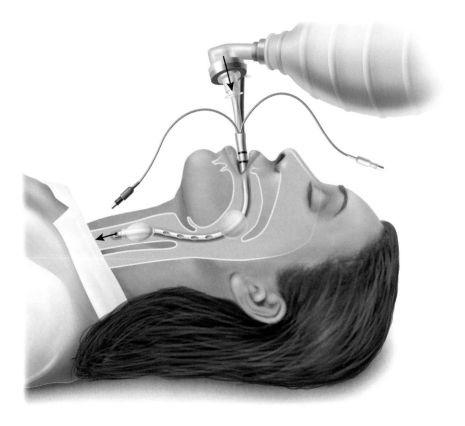

FIGURE 3-11   Combitube, tracheal placement.

airway reflexes when tracheal intubation is not possible. The LMA reduces the risk of aspiration as compared to ventilating the patient by bag-mask alone.

Insert the laryngeal mask airway blindly without visualizing the vocal cords (Figure 3-12). To confirm proper placement, ensure that:

- You can't detect air leaks around the cuff of the mask covering the glottic opening.
- Equal breath sounds are heard in both lungs.
- Air movement is unrestricted with compression of the ventilation bag.
- No gastric contents are present in the LMA.

Testing Tips

- You *cannot* administer medications through the Combitube or LMA.

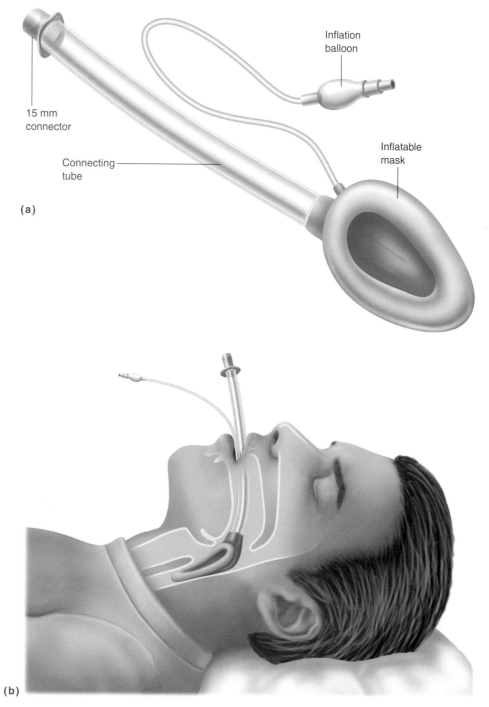

FIGURE 3-12 Laryngeal Mask Airway (LMA). (a) The LMA consists of an inflatable silicone mask and rubber connecting tube. (b) When the mask is inflated, the LMA is pushed up against the tracheal opening and held there, forming a low-pressure seal around the laryngeal inlet.

Algorithm for Respiratory Distress and Arrest

The following algorithm may help you assess patients in respiratory distress with a pulse.

Determine responsiveness

If patient is responsive, able to speak, and ventilating adequately apply supplemental oxygen

If the patient is unresponsive, open the airway using manual maneuvers.

↓

Check for breathing: Look, listen, and feel.

↓

Inadequate breathing or not breathing: Give 2 rescue breaths using a barrier device.

↓

Check for pulse: If present, continue airway assessment.

↓

Reassess for breathing.

↓

Insert oropharyngeal or nasopharyngeal airway.

↓

If the patient is not breathing, deliver one breath every 5–6 seconds (6–7 mL/kg) over 1 second each.

↓

Attempt intubation.
(Have suction available.)

- Take no longer than 30 seconds with each attempt before withdrawing and ventilating the patient.
- Confirm ET tube placement using both clinical means and confirmation devices.

↓

Deliver 1 breath every 6–8 seconds over 1 second each.

↓

If endotracheal intubation is unsuccessful, consider another alternate airway device (LMA or Combitube).

◇ ◇ ◇ **Testing Tips**

- Do not interrupt CPR to insert an advanced airway until absolutely necessary. Have your equipment prepared and the device ready to insert in the patient's mouth before compressions stop. Resume CPR as soon as the device is in place.

The Bottom Line

If you are unable to secure and maintain a patent airway with adequate oxygenation and ventilation, your patient may die. The key to effective management of the airway and ventilation is to move from basic maneuvers to more complex devices and techniques. Coupled with frequent reevaluation, this will ensure that your patient will have enough oxygen and will properly eliminate carbon dioxide so that normal life processes can continue.

4

Public Access Defibrillation

The American Heart Association added public access defibrillation to the 2000 ACLS guidelines to provide a basic understanding of the role of public access defibrillation and the ACLS Chain of Survival. You will find automated external defibrillators in public places such as shopping malls, airports, airplanes, large industrial complexes, schools, and sporting and entertainment arenas. This means that you may have this vital piece of equipment at your disposal to care for victims of cardiac arrest in the out-of-hospital setting (Figure 4-1). Some hospitals have also placed them throughout their clinics, facilities, and even on their code carts so that defibrillation can be provided more quickly than ever before.

During the ACLS course, you may be called on to demonstrate your ability to use an AED safely and efficiently, following the AED Algorithm.

The Basics of Automated External Defibrillators (AEDs)

Automated external defibrillators are very similar in their construction and operation. Though some variability exists, the basic operational procedures are similar enough to allow you to use any of these devices in an emergency situation if you remember the critical steps noted below. After you have determined that your patient is not breathing and has no pulse, have another rescuer begin CPR. Then follow these steps to use an AED:

1. Turn on the AED.
   - This may require you to push a button or merely open the lid of the device.
   - The AED will automatically begin providing you with audible instructions for its use.
   - Begin the next appropriate steps if you know them. You are not required to wait for the machine-generated voice prompts if you are familiar with the AED.

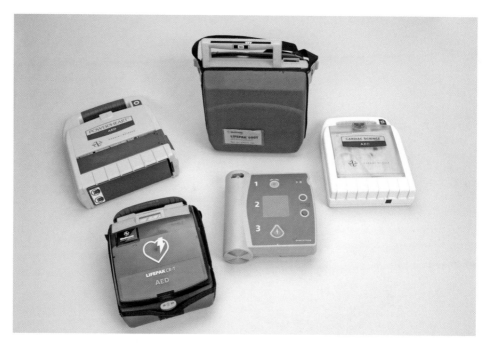

FIGURE 4-1 Automated external defibrilators.

- If there is another rescuer, have him or her continue CPR while you turn on the AED, attach the electrodes, and attach the AED cables. Do not stop CPR until advised to stop by the AED voice prompt.
2. Attach the electrodes to the patient.
   - Most AEDs have electrodes that are prewired to the AED cables, but some older models require you to connect the cables to the electrodes.
   - To assist the lay rescuer, proper placement of the AED electrodes is usually illustrated either on the electrodes themselves or on their packaging (Figure 4-2). Electrode placement is the same as for standard defibrillators.
   - Ensure that the patient's skin is dry. If the patient has excessive chest hair, shave the chest with the razor contained in the AED kit. Try not to nick the skin, because cuts in the skin can cause burns during defibrillation.
3. Attach the AED cables to the AED.
   - Some AEDs have a preconnected cable; others require you to connect the cable to the AED. There is usually a blinking light or some other indicator to show you where to insert the cable connector. Securely fasten the connector into the designated socket.
4. Analyze the heart rhythm for the presence of VF/VT.
   - Some AEDs require you to push a button marked "ANALYZE." Others will automatically analyze the ECG rhythm once the patient is connected to the electrodes and the cable is connected to the AED. Follow the voice prompts if you are not familiar with the AED.

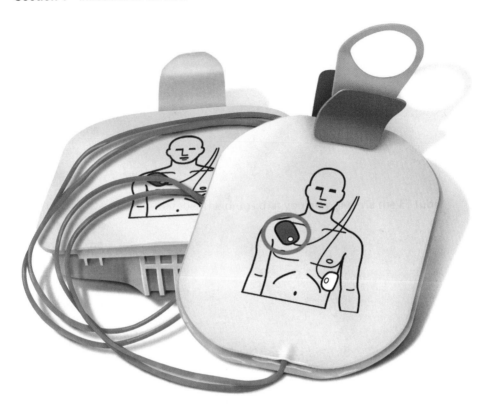

FIGURE 4-2   Correct patch placement is shown on automated external defibrillator pads.

- Some models have a small ECG screen that allows you to see the patient's rhythm. If you see a shockable rhythm, you cannot override the machine and immediately proceed to defibrillate. You must allow the AED to perform the analyze function.
- Stop CPR and do not touch or move the patient during the analyze phase.
- It is helpful to state *"All clear!"* to alert other rescuers not to touch the patient.
- The AED will only detect the presence of VF/VT. Asystole or any other nonshockable rhythm will result in the machine prompting *"No Shock Advised."* If this occurs, begin CPR, starting with chest compressions. Perform 5 cycles of 30 compressions to 2 ventilations, then assess the pulse and analyze the rhythm (older AEDs may require that you analyze after 1 minute).

5. Charge the AED.
   - Most AEDs automatically charge the device if VT or VF is detected. This will be preceded by a voice prompt such as *"Charging! Do not touch the patient!"*
   - Some older models will require you to push a separate button marked "CHARGE," which may be the same button used for both the "ANALYZE" and "SHOCK" functions. Be careful to activate the appropriate button.

6. Defibrillate the patient.
   - Once charged, the device will give a voice instruction such as *"Push to Shock."* Often, the "SHOCK" button will be illuminated or flashing.
   - Announce your intention to defibrillate by stating *"I'm clear, you're clear, everyone is clear!"* while at the same time scanning up and down the patient's body to ensure that no one is touching the patient.
   - Push the appropriate button.

Note: There are still a few AEDs in the community that are fully automatic. They begin the analyze function, charge the AED, and defibrillate the patient without your intervention. They will announce what they are doing and warn you to not touch the patient. Be extremely careful handling the patient, should you encounter such a device!

AED Algorithm

The sequence and prompts in the AED that you encounter may vary. Before the new AHA Guidelines were published in November of 2005, AEDs were programmed to deliver 3 shocks in rapid succession, pausing only to reevaluate the ECG rhythm between shocks. The authors of the new guidelines felt that this sequence resulted in long delays until CPR was performed. The 2005 Guidelines recommend that manufacturers reprogram existing AEDs to deliver 1 shock at a time with a 2-minute pause between shocks so that 5 cycles of CPR can be performed. Until all AEDs are updated, you may encounter either an AED that delivers a 3-shock sequence with a 1-minute pause for CPR, or a new or reprogrammed AED that delivers a 1-shock sequence with a 2-minute pause for CPR. If you are not familiar with the AED you are using, be sure to follow the voice prompts. For the purpose of the algorithm below, "old AED" refers to an AED that is still programmed according to the 2000 Guidelines to deliver shocks in sets of 3 sequences. "New AED" refers to AEDs that are programmed according to the 2005 Guidelines.

▶ Check for patient responsiveness

▶ If unresponsive, call 911

▶ Get the AED if you are alone

▶ Send someone for the AED if you have a partner, and continue your patient assessment

↓

▶ Perform Primary ABCD survey

↓

▶ If the patient is not breathing: Give 2 slow rescue breaths using a barrier device

↓

▶ Check for pulse for 10 seconds

↓

(continued)

▶ If there is no pulse: Start CPR until an AED is available

▶ (30 compressions: 2 ventilations)

▶ If an AED is immediately available: Proceed to AED operation

(If the arrest occurred out-of-hospital, was not witnessed, and no one is performing CPR, continue CPR for 2 minutes before you deliver the first shock)

↓

▶ Attempt defibrillation with the AED if a shock is advised

↓

▶ If *"No Shock Advised"* or after the appropriate number of shock(s) are delivered:

(Old AED: 3 shocks; New AED: 1 shock)

▶ Perform CPR

(Old AED: 1 minute; New AED: 2 minutes)

▶ Provide supplemental oxygen and insert an oropharyngeal airway

↓

▶ Reassess the need to defibrillate by pushing the "ANALYZE" button

▶ Defibrillate again if indicated

(Old AED: Up to 3 shocks; New AED: 1 shock)

↓

▶ Perform CPR

(Old AED: 1 minute; New AED: 2 minutes)

↓

▶ Repeat the sequence of defibrillation and CPR until Advanced Life Support arrives, or reassess if the patient starts to move

◆ ◆ ◆ **Testing Tips**

- Do not place the defibrillation patches over an implanted electronic device (such as a pacemaker).
- Remove any medication patches and wipe the skin before applying defibrillation patches.
- Move your patient away from any standing water and dry off the patient's chest before defibrillation.
- Use the proper CPR technique of 100 compressions per minute and a ratio of 30:2 compressions to breaths.
- Be sure that no one (including you!) is touching the patient when the shock is delivered!
- After each defibrillation, begin with chest compressions.
- Don't forget to use supplemental oxygen and an airway adjunct, if available.
- If additional rescuers assist you, have them take over CPR while you operate the AED.
- Minimize interruptions to CPR.
- Alternate rescuers performing chest compressions to ensure good quality CPR.

The Bottom Line

Using an AED for the first time can be unnerving. You cannot see the ECG tracing, so you must understand that the machine's rhythm analysis system is very accurate. Be patient, because you'll need to wait a few extra seconds while the AED interprets the rhythm. The next time you are at an airport, in a major sports stadium, or at a large shopping center, look around. Make a note of where the AEDs are located so you will be prepared if you need to use one.

5

ECG Rhythms and ACLS Algorithms

> **Interpretation of the ECG rhythm is an important element** in your assessment of patients with emergency cardiac conditions. Look for key features of the ECG that, if abnormal, can significantly impair cardiac output or can signal an impending problem. Assess rate, rhythm, location of impulse origination, and impulse conduction pathway. This interpretation, coupled with your physical assessment of the patient, will help you form a clear clinical picture that will allow you to select the correct treatment plan.

ECG Rhythms

When you interpret a patient's ECG rhythm, you will evaluate its significance based on your clinical exam of the patient. Each rhythm may present with different clinical outcomes:

- Rate and rhythm produce a pulse with adequate perfusion.
- Rate and rhythm produce mechanical action that produces a pulse, but perfusion is inadequate.
- Rate and rhythm are disorganized, or are too fast or too slow, and no effective circulation is produced—there is no pulse.

When you provide Advanced Cardiac Life Support, make prevention of cardiac arrest your highest priority. Intervene aggressively for the patient who has an unstable rhythm with the potential to deteriorate into cardiac arrest.

Hemodynamic Instability

After you interpret an abnormal ECG rhythm, you must decide what treatment path to follow. To determine if the rhythm is stable or unstable, look for serious signs or symptoms that indicate hemodynamic instability. These include:

- Altered mental status
- Chest pain
- Hypotension or clinical signs of shock
- Difficulty breathing with signs of congestive heart failure
- Syncope

 ## ECGs—Bradycardias

Bradycardia is any rhythm that is slower than 60 bpm. The type of bradycardia depends on the origin of the rhythm. You will determine the clinical significance of the rhythm by how slow the rate is and how well the patient tolerates it. For example, a healthy marathon runner may normally have a resting heart rate that is 50 beats per minute or slower, whereas an elderly patient with that same heart rate often has low blood pressure or other signs of shock. First, assess the rhythm to see if it is hemodynamically unstable. Next, interpret the rhythm and look for possible reversible causes of it. Lastly, treat it using the appropriate algorithm.

Sinus Bradycardia

In a sinus bradycardia, impulses originate in the SA node at a slow rate. The onset and termination of the rhythm is gradual and regular. Sinus bradycardia is illustrated in Figure 5-1. The features of this rhythm are listed in Table 5-1.

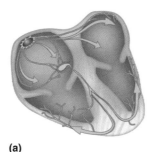

(a)

(b)

FIGURE 5-1   (a) Sinus bradycardia originates from the SA node. (b) Sinus bradycardia.

TABLE 5-1   Sinus Bradycardia

Rhythm	Regular
Rate	< 60 bpm
P wave	■ One before each QRS ■ Normal size and shape
PR interval	0.12–0.20
QRS	≤0.12 sec in the absence of an intraventricular conduction delay
Common causes	■ Normal for physically fit adults ■ Medications (e.g., calcium channel blockers, beta-blockers, digoxin, CNS depressants) ■ Vagus nerve stimulation (e.g., gagging, vomiting, carotid massage) ■ Acute coronary syndrome (ACS) that affects circulation to the SA node (right coronary artery); often, inferior MI ■ Hypoxia ■ Hypothermia
Signs and symptoms	■ Fatigue ■ Dizziness or lightheadedness ■ Weakness ■ Syncope ■ Hypotension ■ Shortness of breath ■ Congestive heart failure (CHF) ■ Chest pressure, tightness, and/or pain
Management	If the patient is symptomatic due to a slow rate, follow the Bradycardia Algorithm.

Junctional Rhythm

In a junctional rhythm, impulses originate in the AV junction in a retrograde (backward) and antegrade (forward) direction. Junctional rhythm is illustrated in Figure 5-2. The features of this rhythm are listed in Table 5-2.

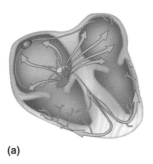

(a)

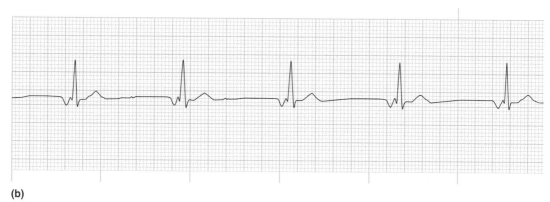

(b)

FIGURE 5-2 (a) Junctional escape rhythms originate in the AV node. (b) Junctional rhythm.

TABLE 5-2 **Junctional Rhythm**

Rhythm	Regular
Rate	40–60 bpm
P wave	▪ May precede, coincide with, or follow the QRS ▪ If seen, will be inverted in leads II, III, and aVF ▪ Normal size and shape
PR interval	< 0.12 sec if P wave is present before the QRS complex
QRS	≤ 0.12 sec in the absence of an intraventricular conduction delay
Common causes	▪ Digitalis intoxication ▪ Vagal stimulation ▪ Heart disease

(continued)

Signs and symptoms	■ Fatigue ■ Dizziness or lightheadedness ■ Weakness ■ Syncope ■ Hypotension ■ Shortness of breath ■ Congestive heart failure ■ Chest pressure, tightness, and/or pain
Management	If the patient is symptomatic due to a slow rate, follow the Bradycardia Algorithm.

Ventricular Escape Rhythm (Idioventricular Rhythm)

A ventricular escape rhythm, which is also called an idioventricular rhythm, results if the SA and AV nodes fail to depolarize or if conduction through the bundle of His is blocked. Because the rate associated with this rhythm is very slow, your patient will usually have very serious signs or symptoms. Prepare for external cardiac pacing. Ventricular escape rhythm is illustrated in Figure 5-3. The features of this rhythm are listed in Table 5-3.

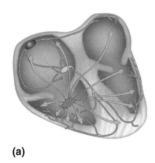

(a)

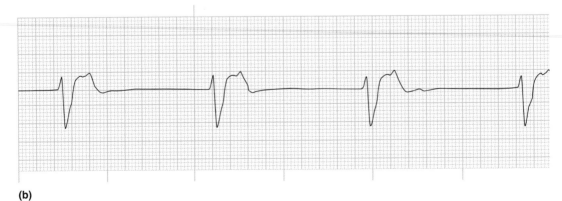

(b)

FIGURE 5-3   (a) Ventricular escape rhythm originates from a single site in the ventricle. (b) Ventricular escape rhythm.

TABLE 5-3   **Ventricular Escape Rhythm (Idioventricular Rhythm)**

Rhythm	Regular to slightly irregular
Rate	20–40 bpm
P wave	■ Usually absent ■ If present, not associated with the QRS complex
PR interval	Absent
QRS	≤ 0.12 sec
Common causes	■ Failure of the SA node ■ Failure of the AV junction ■ Metabolic imbalances ■ Digoxin toxicity
Signs and symptoms	■ Fatigue ■ Dizziness or lightheadedness ■ Weakness ■ Syncope ■ Hypotension ■ Shortness of breath ■ Congestive heart failure ■ Chest pressure, tightness, and/or pain
Management	If the patient is symptomatic due to a slow rate, follow the Bradycardia Algorithm.

First-Degree AV Block

In first-degree AV block, the impulse originates in the SA node and is conducted to the ventricles, but there is a consistent delay in conduction (partial block) at the AV junction. This rhythm does not cause symptoms unless the underlying ventricular rate is slow. First-degree AV block is illustrated in Figure 5-4. The features of this rhythm are listed in Table 5-4.

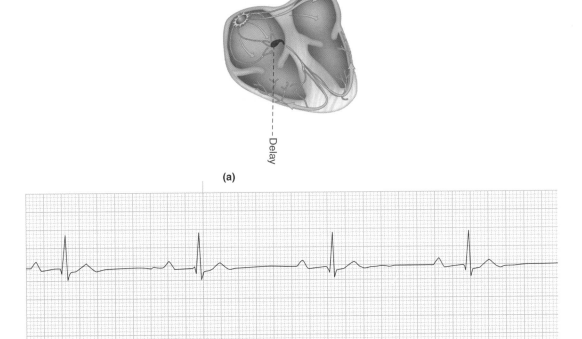

Delay

(a)

(b)

FIGURE 5-4   (a) In first-degree AV heart block, impulses originate in the SA node but are delayed in the AV node. (b) First-degree AV block.

TABLE 5-4   **First-Degree AV Block**

Rhythm	Regular or irregular
Rate	Dependent on the underlying rhythm
P wave	■ One before each QRS complex ■ Normal size and shape
PR interval	> 0.20 sec
QRS	≤ 0.12 sec in the absence of an intraventricular conduction delay
Common causes	■ Normal variant ■ AV node ischemia ■ Cardiac medications, including digoxin, beta-blockers, and calcium channel blockers ■ ACS that affects circulation to the SA node (right coronary artery), most often inferior MI

Signs and symptoms	▪ Usually asymptomatic unless associated with an underlying bradycardia
Management	If the rate is slow and the patient is symptomatic, follow the Bradycardia Algorithm.

Type I Second-Degree AV Block (Mobitz Type I; Wenckebach)

In type I second-degree AV block, which is also referred to as a Mobitz type I or Wenckebach, the impulse originates in the SA node and is increasingly slowed, resulting in progressive lengthening of the PR interval until a sinus impulse is not conducted due to the refractory state of the bundle of His. This results in a dropped QRS complex. Type I second-degree AV block is illustrated in Figure 5-5. The features of this rhythm are listed in Table 5-5.

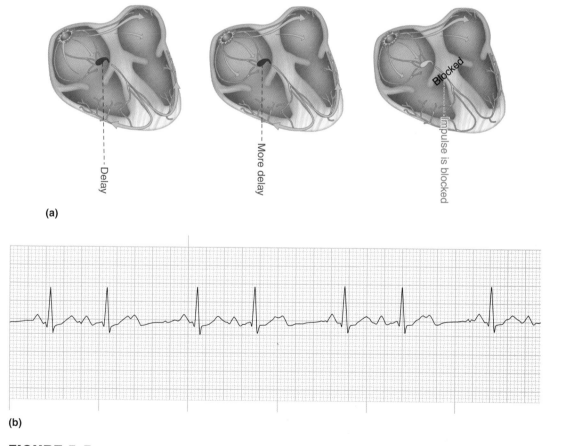

(a)

(b)

FIGURE 5-5 (a) In type I second-degree heart block, impulses originate in the SA node and are progressively delayed in the AV node until a beat is dropped. (b) Type I second-degree AV block.

TABLE 5-5 Type I Second-Degree AV Block (Mobitz Type I; Wenckebach)

Rhythm	Atrial—regular; ventricular—irregular
Rate	Ventricular rate is slower than the atrial rate
P wave	■ Normal size and shape ■ An occasional P wave is not followed by a QRS complex
PR interval	Progressive lengthening until a P wave is not followed by a QRS complex
QRS	≤ 0.12 sec in the absence of an intraventricular conduction delay
Common causes	■ Cardiac medications, including digoxin, beta-blockers, and calcium channel blockers ■ ACS that affects circulation to the SA node (right coronary artery), most often inferior MI
Signs and symptoms	■ Fatigue ■ Dizziness or lightheadedness ■ Weakness ■ Syncope ■ Hypotension ■ Shortness of breath ■ Congestive heart failure ■ Chest pressure, tightness, and/or pain
Management	If the patient is symptomatic due to a slow rate, follow the Bradycardia Algorithm.

Type II Second-Degree AV Block (Mobitz Type II)

In type II second-degree AV block (Mobitz type II), most impulses originating in the SA node are conducted to the ventricles, but there is a periodic, suddenly dropped QRS complex without prior lengthening of the PR interval. Be prepared to apply external pacing if your patient presents with this rhythm. Type II second-degree AV block is illustrated in Figure 5-6. The features of this rhythm are listed in Table 5-6.

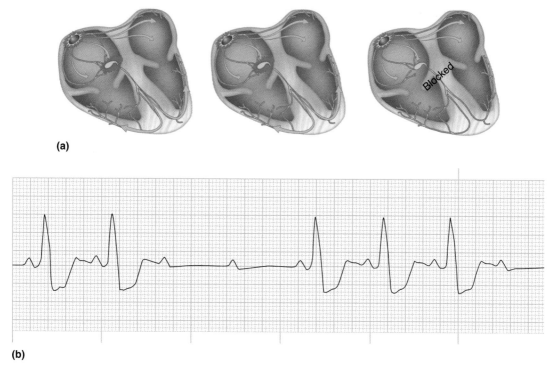

(a)

(b)

FIGURE 5-6   (a) In type II second-degree heart block, impulses originate in the SA node. Some of them are blocked in the AV node. (b) Type II second-degree AV block.

TABLE 5-6   Type II Second-Degree AV Block (Mobitz Type II)

Rhythm	Atrial—regular; ventricular—irregular
Rate	Ventricular rate is slower than the atrial rate
P wave	■ Normal size and shape ■ An occasional P wave not followed by a QRS complex
PR interval	May be < or > 0.20 sec, but will remain the same where P waves precede QRS complexes
QRS	Usually > 0.12 sec
Common causes	■ Anterior MI ■ Degenerative conduction changes
Signs and symptoms	■ Fatigue ■ Dizziness or lightheadedness ■ Weakness ■ Syncope ■ Hypotension ■ Shortness of breath ■ Congestive heart failure ■ Chest pressure, tightness, and/or pain
Management	If the patient is symptomatic due to a slow rate, follow the Bradycardia Algorithm.

Third-Degree AV Block (Complete Heart Block)

In third-degree AV block (complete heart block), the atria and ventricles depolarize independently. Impulses originating in the SA node may be blocked at the AV node or the bundle of His, or at the bundle branches. Many patients with third-degree AV block are clinically unstable. Be prepared for external pacing. Third-degree AV block is illustrated in Figure 5-7. The features of this rhythm are listed in Table 5-7.

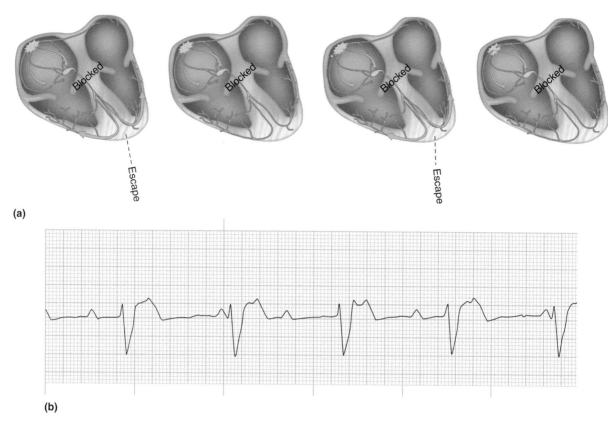

(a)

(b)

FIGURE 5-7 (a) In third-degree AV block, the impulses that originate in the SA node are completely blocked at the AV node. The ventricles are depolarized by an escape pacemaker in the AV node, HIS bundle, or bundle branches. (b) Third-degree AV block.

TABLE 5-7 **Third-Degree AV Block (Complete Heart Block)**

Rhythm	Atrial—regular; ventricular—regular
Rate	Ventricular rate depends on the source of the escape pacemaker (usually very slow); atrial rate is usually 60–100 bpm
P wave	■ Normal size and shape ■ No association between the P waves and the QRS complexes (atrial-ventricular dissociation)
PR interval	None (atrial and ventricles are independent of each other)
QRS	Narrow (≤ 0.12 sec) or wide (≥ 0.12 sec) (more common)

(continued)

Common causes	■ Acute myocardial infarction
	■ Toxic levels of medications, such as beta-blockers, calcium channel blockers, or digitalis
	■ Damage to the AV node or bundle branches
Signs and symptoms	■ Fatigue
	■ Dizziness or lightheadedness
	■ Weakness
	■ Syncope
	■ Hypotension
	■ Shortness of breath
	■ Congestive heart failure
	■ Chest pressure, tightness, and/or pain
Management	If the patient is symptomatic due to a slow rate, follow the Bradycardia Algorithm.

Bradycardia Algorithm

▶ Primary ABCD survey

▶ Secondary ABCD survey

▶ O₂; IV; cardiac monitor; assess vital signs; attach pulse oximeter; obtain history, physical exam, 12-lead ECG, and portable chest X-ray

▶ Are serious signs and symptoms present due to the bradycardia? (Chest pain, shortness of breath, decreased level of consciousness, hypotension, shock, pulmonary congestion, CHF, acute MI)

▶ If serious signs and symptoms present:
Prepare for transcutaneous pacing

▶ Consider atropine, 0.5 mg IVP; may repeat every 3–5 minutes up to 3 mg (total dose)
(While waiting to begin pacing)

↓

▶ Initiate transcutaneous pacing (TCP)
(Do not delay TCP to start IV or while waiting for atropine to take effect.)
Use immediately for Type II second-degree AV block or third-degree AV block.

↓

If transcutaneous pacing is ineffective or unavailable, consider the following until transvenous pacing is available:

- Dopamine IV infusion, 2–10 mcg/kg/min
    OR
- Epinephrine IV infusion, 2–10 mcg/min
    OR
- Isoproterenol infusion, 2–10 mcg/min (if transplanted heart or for beta-blocker overdose)

◇ ◇ ◇ **Testing Tips**

- If bradycardia is stable, observe the patient and reassess often.
- Atropine is not effective for infranodal block. If this block is present, prepare to pace immediately.
- Some patients are bradycardic secondary to hypoxia. Ensure adequate oxygenation and ventilation.

ECGs—Tachycardias

When you treat tachycardia, consider whether the patient is hemodynamically compromised. If the patient's heart rate is greater than 150 bpm, the patient is more likely to be unstable.

Narrow-Complex Tachycardias

Narrow-complex tachycardias, also called supraventricular tachycardias (SVTs), include:

- Sinus tachycardia
- Atrial tachycardia
- Junctional tachycardia
- Multifocal atrial tachycardia
- Atrial flutter
- Atrial fibrillation

Sinus Tachycardia

In sinus tachycardia, impulses originate in the SA node at a rapid rate. This rhythm usually occurs in response to an injury, illness, or stressor. Sinus tachycardia also occurs after stimulants are used. Sinus tachycardia is illustrated in Figure 5-8. The features of this rhythm are provided in Table 5-8.

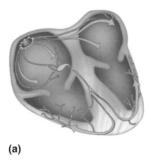

(a)

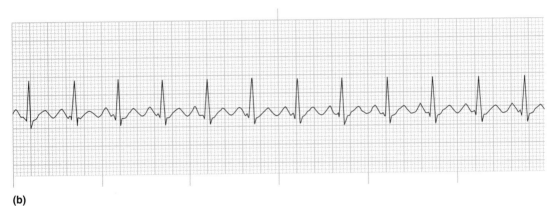

(b)

FIGURE 5-8 (a) In sinus tachycardia, impulses originate in the SA node and follow normal conduction pathways. (b) Sinus tachycardia.

TABLE 5-8 Sinus Tachycardia

Rhythm	Regular
Rate	> 100 bpm
P wave	■ One before each QRS complex ■ Normal size and shape
PR interval	0.12–0.20 sec
QRS	≤ 0.12 sec in the absence of an intraventricular conduction delay
Common causes	■ Fever ■ Exercise ■ Pain ■ Hypovolemia ■ AMI ■ Hypoxia ■ Shock ■ Anxiety ■ Hyperthyroidism ■ Stimulant use (caffeine, cocaine, methamphetamine, etc.)
Signs and symptoms	If signs and symptoms are present, they are due to the cause of the tachycardia, such as fever, pain, anxiety, etc.
Management	Treat the underlying cause of the tachycardia.

Atrial Tachycardia

Atrial tachycardia is illustrated in Figure 5-9. The features of this rhythm are listed in Table 5-9. Paroxysmal atrial tachycardia (PAT), which is atrial tachycardia that begins or ends suddenly, is illustrated in Figure 5-9c. Another narrow-complex tachycardia that is often difficult to distinguish from PAT, and is treated emergently the same is AV nodal reentrant tachycardia.

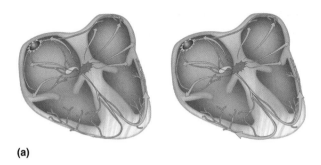

(a)

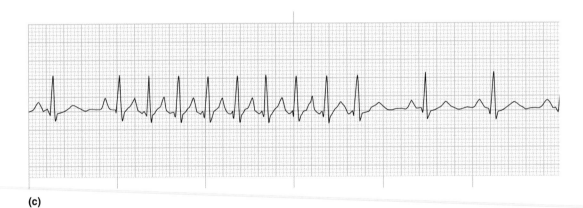

(b)

(c)

FIGURE 5-9 (a) Atrial tachycardia originates from a single site in the atrium. (b) Atrial tachycardia. (c) Paroxysmal atrial tachycardia.

TABLE 5-9 Atrial Tachycardia

Rhythm	Regular
Rate	150–250 bpm
P wave	Not readily seen because they are buried in the T wave of the preceding beat
PR interval	0.12–0.20 sec if P wave visible
QRS	≤ 0.12 sec in the absence of an intraventricular conduction delay
Common causes	▪ May occur in healthy persons due to physical or psychological stress, hypoxia, sleep deprivation, electrolyte imbalances, caffeine, nicotine, marijuana, or many medications ▪ More commonly occurs in patients with an accessory conduction pathway, coronary artery disease (CAD), chronic obstructive pulmonary disease (COPD), or congestive heart failure (CHF)
Signs and symptoms	▪ Palpitations ▪ Anxiety ▪ Dyspnea ▪ Lightheadedness ▪ Weakness ▪ Chest pain or pressure ▪ Nausea ▪ Diaphoresis ▪ Dizziness ▪ Syncope ▪ Possible signs of shock, depending on the duration and rate of the tachycardia
Management	If symptomatic due to a rapid rate, follow the Algorithm for Regular Narrow-Complex Tachycardia.

Junctional Tachycardia

In a junctional tachycardia, impulses originate in the AV junction with transmission in a retrograde (backward) and antegrade (forward) direction. Junctional tachycardia is relatively unusual—try to determine the cause if you detect it. Junctional tachycardia is illustrated in Figure 5-10. The features of this rhythm are listed in Table 5-10.

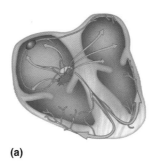

(a)

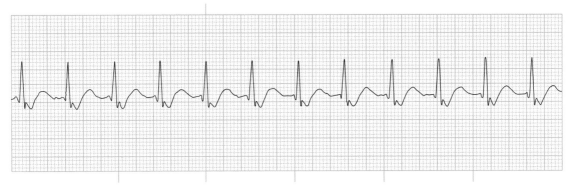

(b)

FIGURE 5-10 (a) Junctional tachycardia originates from a single focus in the AV node. (b) Junctional tachycardia.

TABLE 5-10 **Junctional Tachycardia**

Rhythm	Regular
Rate	100–180 bpm
P wave	■ May precede, coincide with, or follow the QRS complex ■ If seen, will be inverted in leads II, III, and aVF ■ Normal size and shape
PR interval	< 0.12 sec if P wave present before the QRS complex
QRS	≤ 0.12 sec in the absence of an intraventricular conduction delay
Common causes	■ Digitalis intoxication ■ Heart disease ■ Consequence of ACS

Signs and symptoms	■ Fatigue ■ Dizziness or lightheadedness ■ Weakness ■ Syncope ■ Hypotension ■ Shortness of breath ■ Chest pressure, tightness, and/or pain
Management	If the patient is symptomatic due to a rapid rate, follow the Algorithm for Regular Narrow-Complex Tachycardia. Cardioversion is not recommended.

Multifocal Atrial Tachycardia (MAT)

In multifocal atrial tachycardia (MAT), impulses originate irregularly and rapidly at different points in the atria. Multifocal atrial tachycardia is illustrated in Figure 5-11. The features of this rhythm are listed in Table 5-11.

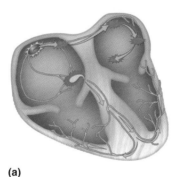

(a)

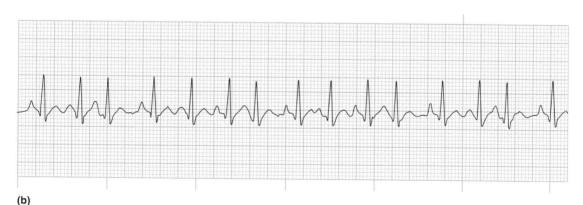

(b)

FIGURE 5-11   (a) In multifocal atrial tachycardia, each heartbeat originates from a different focus in the atria. (b) Multifocal atrial tachycardia.

TABLE 5-11   **Multifocal Atrial Tachycardia (MAT)**

Rhythm	Irregular
Rate	> 100 bpm
P wave	Three or more P waves of varying size, shape, and direction are required for a diagnosis of MAT
PR interval	Variable
QRS	≤ 0.12 sec in the absence of an intraventricular conduction delay
Common causes	■ COPD is the most common cause ■ ACS ■ Hypoxia ■ Digoxin toxicity ■ Hypokalemia ■ Hypomagnesemia
Signs and symptoms	The patient may be asymptomatic. If signs and symptoms are present, they can include: ■ Fatigue ■ Dizziness or lightheadedness ■ Weakness ■ Syncope ■ Hypotension ■ Shortness of breath ■ Chest pressure, tightness, and/or pain
Management	If symptomatic due to a rapid rate, follow the Algorithm for Regular Narrow-Complex Tachycardia. Cardioversion is not recommended.

Algorithm for Regular Narrow-Complex Tachycardia Algorithm

▶ Primary ABCD survey

↓

▶ O₂; IV; cardiac monitor; assess vital signs; attach pulse oximeter; obtain history, physical exam, 12-lead ECG, and portable chest X-ray

↓

▶ If sinus rhythm:
  Treat underlying cause

  ↓

▶ For other hemodynamically stable, regular SVT rhythms with narrow QRS:
  Attempt vagal maneuvers

  ↓

▶ Adenosine 6 mg rapid IVP over 1–3 seconds*
▶ If needed, give adenosine, 12 mg rapid IVP over 1–3 seconds after 1–2 minutes
▶ May repeat adenosine 12 mg dose once in 1–2 minutes

  ↓

▶ If SVT persists:
  • Consider diltiazem
        OR
  • Beta-blockers (cautiously if CHF or pulmonary disease)
▶ *If hemodynamically unstable with ventricular rate > 150 bpm:*
  • Immediate synchronized cardioversion 50 (PSVT and atrial flutter only)
    100–200–300–360 J (or equivalent biphasic dose)

*If the patient is taking dipyridamole or carbamazepine, reduce the dose of adenisone to 3 mg.

◇ ◇ ◇ Testing Tips

  ▪ After choosing an antiarrhythmic agent, continue to administer it until you have reached the maximum dose or the patient develops complications. Then move to another agent or consider cardioversion.
  ▪ Do not cardiovert junctional tachycardia, multifocal atrial tachycardia, or sinus tachycardia.
  ▪ Cardioversion is only for the unstable patient who is not tolerating the tachycardia.
  ▪ Administer analgesics and/or sedation to conscious patients before cardioversion if time permits.

Atrial Flutter and Fibrillation

Atrial flutter and atrial fibrillation originate in the atria. The atrial rate in both of these rhythms is very rapid; however, the ventricular rate will vary. Patients are most likely to have signs and symptoms related to atrial flutter and fibrillation if there is a rapid ventricular response.

Atrial Flutter

In atrial flutter, impulses travel in a circular pattern in the atria. Because the AV node often blocks the conduction of atrial impulses in a fixed ratio, it is not common to see a ventricular rate of 150 bpm (2:1 conduction) or 75 bpm (4:1 conduction). Atrial flutter is illustrated in Figure 5-12. The features of this rhythm are listed in Table 5-12.

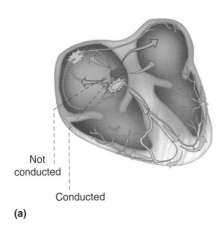

Not
conducted

Conducted

(a)

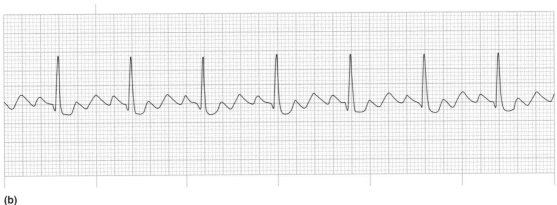

(b)

FIGURE 5-12   (a) In atrial flutter, impulses fire at 250-350 bpm from an ectopic site in the atria. Some of the impulses are blocked at the AV node. (b) Atrial flutter.

TABLE 5-12   Atrial Flutter

Rhythm	Atrial—regular; ventricular—often regular, but may be irregular
Rate	Atrial rate 220–350 bpm (often 300 bpm); ventricular response variable but usually < 180 bpm due to the limits of AV node conduction

P wave	■ No identifiable P waves
	■ Flutter waves present in "sawtooth" or "picket fence" pattern
PR interval	Cannot be measured
QRS	≤ 0.12 sec in the absence of an intraventricular conduction delay
Common causes	■ Hypoxia
	■ Pulmonary embolism
	■ ACS
	■ CAD
	■ CHF
	■ Digitalis or quinidine toxicity
	■ Mitral or tricuspid valve disease
	■ Cardiac surgery
Signs and symptoms	The patient may be asymptomatic if the ventricular rate is within the normal range. If the ventricular rate is rapid, the patient may exhibit signs and symptoms due to the tachycardia, including:
	■ Palpitations
	■ Fatigue
	■ Dizziness or lightheadedness
	■ Weakness
	■ Syncope
	■ Hypotension
	■ Shortness of breath
	■ Chest pressure, tightness, and/or pain
Management	If symptomatic due to a rapid ventricular response, follow the Algorithm for Atrial Fibrillation and Atrial Flutter with Rapid Narrow-Complex Ventricular Response.

Atrial Fibrillation

In atrial fibrillation, impulses travel in chaotic, random pathways within the atria. Atrial fibrillation is characterized by its irregularly, irregular rhythm. The AV node will allow only some of these impulses through to the ventricle, which will determine the ventricular rate. If the atrial fibrillation is controlled with drugs, the heart rate will be less than 100 bpm. If the atrial fibrillation is uncontrolled and the ventricular rate is very fast, the patient may have life-threatening signs and symptoms. Atrial fibrillation is illustrated in Figure 5-13. The features of this rhythm are listed in Table 5-13.

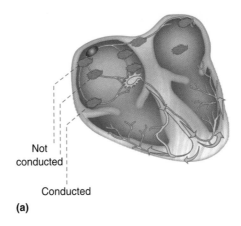

Not
conducted

Conducted

(a)

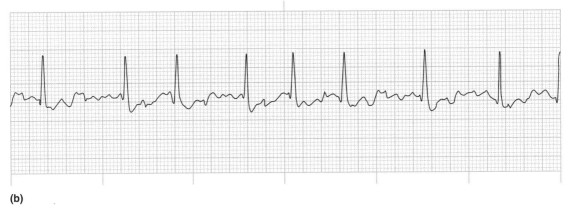

(b)

FIGURE 5-13   (a) In atrial fibrillation, more than 350 impulses originate from random atrial ectopic sites each minute. The AV node blocks some of the impulses. (b) Atrial fibrillation.

TABLE 5-13   Atrial Fibrillation

Rhythm	Irregularly irregular
Rate	Atrial rate usually exceeds 400 bpm; the ventricular response is variable but usually < 180 bpm due to the limits of AV node conduction.
P wave	▪ Absent ▪ Atrial fibrillatory waves present (also called f waves), resulting in a wavering baseline
PR interval	Cannot be measured
QRS	≤ 0.12 sec in the absence of an intraventricular conduction delay

Common causes	■ Hypoxia ■ Pulmonary embolism ■ ACS ■ CAD ■ CHF ■ Cardiomyopathy ■ Digitalis or quinidine toxicity ■ Mitral or tricuspid valve disease ■ Cardiac surgery ■ Pulmonary disease ■ Excessive alcohol consumption ■ Hypokalemia ■ Hypomagnesemia ■ Thyrotoxicosis
Signs and symptoms	The patient may be asymptomatic if the ventricular rate is within the normal range. If the ventricular rate is rapid, the patient may exhibit signs and symptoms due to the tachycardia, including: ■ Fatigue ■ Dizziness or lightheadedness ■ Weakness ■ Syncope ■ Hypotension ■ Shortness of breath ■ Chest pressure, tightness, and/or pain
Management	If the patient is symptomatic due to a rapid ventricular response, follow the Algorithm for Atrial Fibrillation and Atrial Flutter with Rapid Narrow-Complex Ventricular Response.

Algorithm for Atrial Fibrillation and Atrial Flutter with Rapid Narrow-Complex Ventricular Response

▶ Primary ABCD survey

↓

▶ O_2; IV; cardiac monitor; assess vital signs; attach pulse oximeter; obtain history, physical exam, 12-lead ECG, and portable chest X-ray

↓

▶ Is the patient stable but symptomatic?

(continued)

▶ Control rate:
Calcium channel blocker
OR
Beta-blocker (cautiously if CHF or pulmonary disease)

▶ Consider underlying causes

▶ Consult cardiologist

▶ *If hemodynamically unstable with ventricular rate > 150 bpm:*
Immediate synchronized cardioversion
Atrial flutter: 50–100–200–300–360 J (or equivalent biphasic energy)
Atrial fibrillation: 100–200–300–360 J (or equivalent biphasic energy)

Wolff-Parkinson-White (WPW) Syndrome

In patients with Wolff-Parkinson-White (WPW) syndrome, strands of conducting myo-cardial tissue connecting the atria and ventricles persist after birth. This tissue is called an accessory pathway and provides a mechanism for reentry. In WPW, the accessory pathway is able to conduct an impulse from the atria to the ventricles and from the ventricles to the atria. The accessory pathway can conduct impulses from the atrium to the ventricle much faster than is possible through the AV node, resulting in very rapid heart rates. Wolff-Parkinson-White syndrome is illustrated in Figure 5-14. The features of this rhythm are listed in Table 5-14.

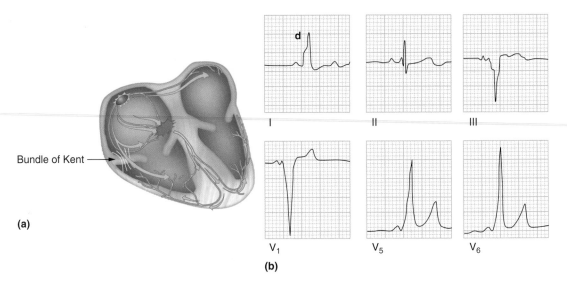

(a)

Bundle of Kent

(b)

FIGURE 5-14   (a) In Wolff-Parkinson-White (WPW) syndrome, impulses travel through an accessory pathway between the atria and ventricles. (b) Wolff-Parkinson-White syndrome. The *"d"* indicates the delta wave.

TABLE 5-14   **Wolff-Parkinson-White (WPW) Syndrome**

Rhythm	Regular
Rate	Usually 60–100 bpm
P wave	One before each QRS; normal size and shape
PR interval	Short (< 0.12 sec)
QRS	Usually > 0.12 sec due to presence of delta wave (slurring of the upstroke of the QRS complex)
Common causes	Congenital in origin
Signs and symptoms	Usually asymptomatic unless a tachycardia develops. If the ventricular rate is rapid, the patient may exhibit signs and symptoms due to the tachycardia, including: ■ Palpitations ■ Fatigue ■ Dizziness or lightheadedness ■ Weakness ■ Syncope ■ Hypotension ■ Shortness of breath ■ Chest pressure, tightness, and/or pain
Management	If symptomatic due to a rapid ventricular response, follow the Algorithm for Wolff-Parkinson-White (WPW) Syndrome with Rapid Ventricular Response.
Notes	WPW is a type of pre-excitation syndrome. "Pre-excitation" refers to rhythms that originate above the ventricles, but the electrical impulse travels to the ventricles using an abnormal pathway (that is, it bypasses the AV node and bundle of His). The ECG hallmarks of WPW syndrome are a short PR interval, a delta wave, and a wide QRS complex.

Algorithm for Wolff-Parkinson-White (WPW) Syndrome with Rapid Ventricular Response

▶ Primary ABCD survey

↓

▶ O$_2$; IV; cardiac monitor; assess vital signs; attach pulse oximeter; obtain history, physical exam, 12-lead ECG, and portable chest X-ray

↓

▶ If hemodynamically stable:
Amiodarone 150 mg IV over 10 minutes

↓

▶ Consult cardiologist
May consider procainamide

↓

▶ *If hemodynamically unstable with ventricular rate > 150 bpm:*
Immediate synchronized cardioversion 100–200–300–360 J (or equivalent biphasic energy)

◇ ◇ ◇ Testing Tips

- Drugs that can be harmful for the patient with WPW include adenosine, beta-blockers, calcium channel blockers, and digoxin.

Ventricular Tachycardia

Impulse conduction is altered in areas of the myocardium affected by ischemia, injury, or infarction. These areas are frequently the source of ectopic impulses that can lead to reentry and a pattern of rapid, repetitive ventricular depolarization, causing ventricular tachycardia.

Ventricular Tachycardia (Monomorphic)

The patient with monomorphic ventricular tachycardia may be stable, hemodynamically unstable, or pulseless and in cardiac arrest. Monomorphic ventricular tachycardia is illustrated in Figure 5-15. The features of this rhythm are listed in Table 5-15.

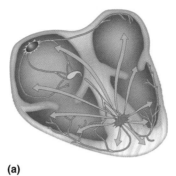

(a)

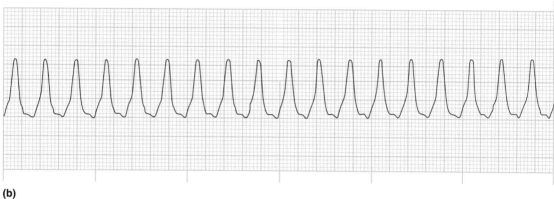

(b)

FIGURE 5-15 (a) Monomorphic ventricular tachycardia originates from a single focus in the ventricle. (b) Ventricular tachycardia (monomorphic).

TABLE 5-15 **Ventricular Tachycardia (Monomorphic)**

Rhythm	Usually regular but may be irregular
Rate	> 100 bpm and usually not > 250 bpm
P wave	Dissociated P waves may be visible
PR interval	Indeterminate
QRS	≥ 0.12 sec
Common causes	■ Usually associated with CAD ■ Can be triggered by electrolyte imbalance or the use of sympathomimetic agents

(continued)

Signs and symptoms	The patient may be asymptomatic, stable but symptomatic, unstable, or pulseless. Symptoms include: ■ Chest pain ■ Palpitations ■ Anxiety ■ Diaphoresis ■ Hypotension ■ Mental status changes ■ Cardiac arrest
Management	Pulseless—see Algorithm for Pulseless VT/VF. Stable or unstable with a pulse—see monomorphic VT algorithm.
Notes	A run of VT is 3 or more sequential PVCs at a rate > 100 bpm. Sustained VT occurs when the rhythm lasts > 30 seconds. Nonsustained VT persists for < 30 seconds.

Algorithm for Ventricular Tachycardia (Monomorphic)

▶ Primary ABCD survey

⬇

▶ O₂; IV; cardiac monitor; assess vital signs; attach pulse oximeter; obtain history, physical exam, 12-lead ECG, and portable chest X-ray

⬇

▶ *If hemodynamically stable:*
Amiodarone, 150 mg IV over 10 minutes; may repeat in 10 minutes if needed; max dose 2.2 g IV/24 hours (1 mg/min infusion for 6 hours; Followed by 0.5 mg/min. infusion for 18 hours)
          OR
If amiodarone is not available:
Lidocaine, 0.5–0.75 mg/kg IVP (up to 1.0–1.5 mg/kg may be given as initial dose)
May repeat with 0.5–0.75 mg/kg every 5–10 minutes; max dose 3 mg/kg
Prepare for elective synchronized cardioversion

⬇

▶ *If hemodynamically unstable with ventricular rate > 150 bpm:*
Immediate synchronized cardioversion 100–200–300–360 J (or equivalent biphasic energy)

↓

▶ *If pulseless:*
Immediate defibrillation: biphasic 120–200 J or monophasic 360 J
Follow the Algorithm for Pulseless VT/VF

◇ ◇ ◇ **Testing Tips**

- After choosing an antiarrhythmic agent, continue to administer it until the rhythm converts, you have reached the maximum dose, or the patient develops complications (such as hypotension or another arrhythmia). Then move to another agent or consider cardioversion.
- The dose of amiodarone is different for the treatment of arrhythmias than it is for VT in cardiac arrest: 150 mg IV over 10 minutes for arrhythmia and 300 mg IVP in cardiac arrest.
- If time and the patient's condition permit, administer sedation before cardioversion.

Ventricular Tachycardia (Polymorphic)

In polymorphic ventricular tachycardia, impulse conduction is slowed in multiple areas affected by ischemia, injury, or infarction. These areas are frequently the source of multiple ectopic (i.e., polymorphic) impulses that travel in a circular pattern and lead to reentry and a pattern of rapid, repetitive ventricular depolarization. Polymorphic ventricular tachycardia is illustrated in Figure 5-16. The features of this rhythm are listed in Table 5-16.

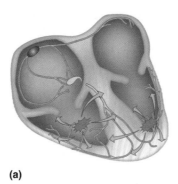

(a)

(b)

FIGURE 5-16   (a) In polymorphic ventricular tachycardia, impulses originate from more than one focus in the ventricles. (b) Ventricular tachycardia (polymorphic).

TABLE 5-16   **Ventricular Tachycardia (Polymorphic)**

Rhythm	Atrial—cannot be determined; ventricular—irregular
Rate	Atrial rate cannot be determined; ventricular rate 150–250 bpm
P wave	Absent
PR interval	Absent
QRS	Vary in size, shape, and amplitude
Common causes	■ CAD ■ Acute myocardial infarction ■ Myocarditis ■ Electrolyte imbalance

Signs and symptoms	■ Chest pain ■ Palpitations ■ Anxiety ■ Hypotension ■ Dizziness ■ Syncope ■ Shortness of breath ■ Mental status changes ■ Cardiac arrest
Management	Pulseless—see the Algorithm for Pulseless VT/VF. Stable or unstable—See the Algorithm for Ventricular Tachycardia (Polymorphic).
Notes	Torsades de pointes (TdP) is a type of polymorphic VT most often seen in the setting of a long QT syndrome due to antiarrhythmic medications or related to a congenital cause.

Algorithm for Ventricular Tachycardia (Polymorphic)

▶ Primary ABCD survey

↓

▶ O_2; IV; cardiac monitor; assess vital signs; attach pulse oximeter; obtain history, physical exam, 12-lead ECG, and portable chest X-ray

↓

▶ Consult expert early

↓

▶ *Normal QT interval and hemodynamically stable:*
Amiodarone, 150 mg IV over 10 minutes; may repeat every 10 minutes if needed; max dose 2.2 g IV/24 hours (1 mg/min. infusion for 6 hours; Followed by 0.5 mg/min. infusion for 18 hours)
        OR
Lidocaine, 0.5–0.75 mg/kg IVP (up to 1.0–1.5 mg/kg may be given as initial dose)

↓

▶ *Prolonged QT interval and hemodynamically stable:*
Correct the causes

(continued)

(Stop drugs that prolong the QT interval; correct electrolyte imbalance; treat the effects of drug overdose)
Infuse magnesium sulfate 1–2 g over 5–60 minutes
With expert advice, consider isoproterenol or overdrive pacing

↓

▶ *If hemodynamically unstable:*
Immediate defibrillation: biphasic 120–200 J or monophasic 360 J

↓

▶ *If pulseless:*
Immediate defibrillation: biphasic 120–200 J or monophasic 360 J
Follow Algorithm for Pulseless VT/VF

Cardiac Arrest Rhythms and Algorithms

Most cardiac arrest victims will have one of three rhythms: (1) ventricular tachycardia (VT or v-tach), (2) ventricular fibrillation (VF or v-fib), or (3) asystole. Experts suspect that most cardiac arrests begin with ventricular ectopy that causes VT. The ventricular tachycardia may initially produce a pulse, but often changes quickly into pulseless VT. As the ischemia worsens, the rhythm further deteriorates into VF. Ventricular fibrillation causes chaotic contraction of the ventricles that does not produce coordinated pumping of the heart and is always without a pulse. Eventually, the acidosis and ischemia worsen until all electrical activity in the heart stops and the patient develops asystole.

Another condition that will result in cardiac arrest is pulseless electrical activity (PEA). While this condition is not a specific rhythm disturbance, PEA is presented here with the other cardiac arrest rhythms because the approach to it is similar to the general treatment of the patient in cardiac arrest.

Rhythm characteristics for ventricular tachycardia have already been presented with the tachycardic rhythms. VT may remain stable or unstable for a period of time or rapidly deteriorate into a pulseless rhythm. Your treatment of VT will depend on the patient's clinical signs and symptoms. Management of pulseless ventricular tachycardia will be discussed in this section.

◆ ◆ ◆ **Testing Tips**

When treating a patient in cardiac arrest:

- Confirm proper endotracheal tube placement and/or adequate ventilation if a nonvisualized airway is used.
- Consider the tracheal tube route for medications until IV or IO access is secured.
- Do not use the Combitube or LMA as a route to administer medications.
- If the patient is successfully resuscitated from ventricular fibrillation or ventricular tachycardia and an antiarrhythmic agent was given, institute a constant maintenance infusion of that agent. If an antiarrhythmic was not given but the initial or subsequent rhythms would have been candidates for antiarrhythmic therapy, administer one-half the usual loading dose and start a continuous infusion (refer to Appendix A for infusion details).
- Continuously monitor CPR to ensure it is being performed with minimal interruption at 100 compressions per minute at a depth of 11/2 to 2 inches.
- Rotate rescuers performing chest compressions often.
- Think of the 6 "Hs" and 6 "Ts" to search for causes of the arrest and treat the specific cause if found:

Hypovolemia	**T**ablet/toxins (overdose)
Hypoxia	**T**amponade (cardiac)
Hydrogen ion (acidosis)	**T**ension pneumothorax
Hypo/hyperkalemia	**T**hrombosis (cardiac)
Hypoglycemia	**T**hrombosis (pulmonary)
Hypothermia	**T**rauma

Ventricular Fibrillation (VF)

Ventricular fibrillation is chaotic ventricular depolarization. It is illustrated in Figure 5-17. The features of this rhythm are provided in Table 5-17.

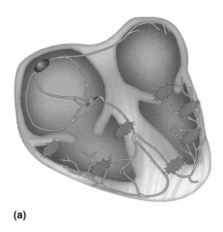

(a)

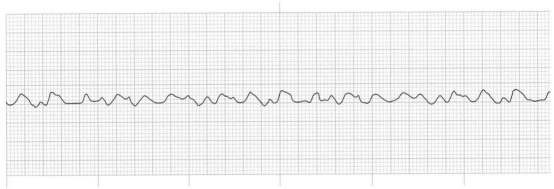

(b)

FIGURE 5-17   (a) During ventricular fibrillation, chaotic electrical activity originates from the ventricles.
(b) Ventricular fibrillation.

TABLE 5-17   Ventricular Fibrillation (VF)

Rhythm	Irregular, chaotic
Rate	Rapid, disorganized
P wave	Absent
PR interval	Absent
QRS	Indistinct; undulations < 3 mm = fine VF; undulations > 3 mm = coarse VF

Common causes	■ Hypoxia
	■ R-on-T premature ventricular contractions (PVCs)
	■ Electrolyte or acid-base imbalance
	■ Medications that prolong the QT interval
	■ ACS leading to myocardial ischemia
	■ Electrocution
	■ Others
Signs and symptoms	■ Loss of consciousness
	■ Irregular breathing that rapidly results in apnea
	■ No pulse
	■ Absent heart sounds
Management	Algorithm for Pulseless VT/VF

Algorithm for Pulseless VT/VF

▶ Primary ABCD survey

▶ If arrest witnessed, defibrillate immediately

▶ If unwitnessed prehospital arrest, give 5 cycles of CPR before defibrillation

↓

▶ Defibrillate pulseless VT/VF 120–200 J biphasic: 360 J monophasic

↓

▶ Continue CPR for 5 cycles: begin with compressions, intubate when possible, IV
(Reassess rhythm at end of the fifth CPR cycle)

↓

▶ Epinephrine, 1 mg (1:10,000 solution) IVP every 3–5 minutes
(ET dose 2.0–2.5 mg)
(May substitute vasopressin 40 units IV/IO for first or second epinephrine dose)

↓

(continued)

▶ Defibrillate with 120–200 J biphasic (or higher): 360 J monophasic after each 5 cycles of CPR

↓

▶ Amiodarone, 300 mg IVP; may repeat once with 150 mg IVP in 3–5 minutes

▶ *If amiodarone not available:*
Lidocaine, 1.0–1.5 mg/kg IVP (ET dose 2–4 mg/kg); may repeat with 0.5–0.75 mg/kg IVP every 5–10 minutes up to 3 mg/kg

▶ *May consider:*
Magnesium, 1–2 g IV if torsades de pointes or hypomagnesemia

▶ *Consider:*
Treatable causes

▶ Reassess pulse if an organized ECG rhythm is observed

◆ ◆ ◆ Testing Tips

- Clear the patient for defibrillation immediately before shock is given. Resume CPR, beginning with chest compressions, immediately after shock is delivered.
- Drugs should be given without interrupting CPR, either before or after defibrillation.
- Be sure you know whether your defibrillator is monophasic or biphasic, and what energy levels are advised by the manufacturer for defibrillation.
- Minimize interruptions to CPR.

Asystole

Asystole, which is also called ventricular standstill, reflects a cessation of ventricular activity. P waves may be observed at its onset. Asystole is illustrated in Figure 5-18. The features of this rhythm are listed in Table 5-18.

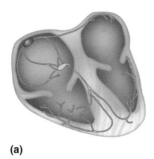

(a)

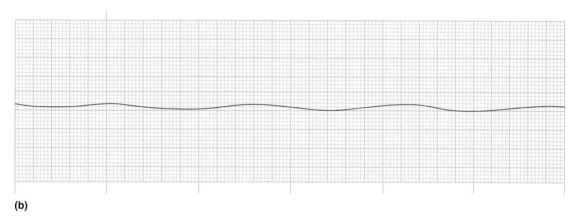

(b)

FIGURE 5-18   (a) During asystole, there is no electrical activity in the heart. (b) Asystole.

TABLE 5-18   **Asystole**

Rhythm	Absent
Rate	Ventricular rate is absent; atrial rate, if present, may be slow or fast
P wave	Usually absent
PR interval	Absent
QRS	Absent

(continued)

Common causes	6 Hs and 6 Ts:
	■ Hypovolemia
	■ Hypoxia
	■ Hydrogen ion (acidosis)
	■ Hypokalemia/hyperkalemia
	■ Hypoglycemia
	■ Hypothermia
	■ Tablets/toxins (overdose)
	■ Tamponade (cardiac)
	■ Tension pneumothorax
	■ Thrombosis (coronary)
	■ Thrombosis (pulmonary)
	■ Trauma
Signs and symptoms	■ Loss of consciousness
	■ Apnea
	■ Lack of pulse
	■ Absent heart sounds
Management	Asystole Algorithm

Asystole Algorithm

▶ Primary ABCD survey, CPR, check ECG rhythm

↓

▶ Confirm asystole: Check lead connections and leads I, II, and III

↓

▶ Check for DNR order and signs of obvious death

↓

▶ Secondary ABCD survey

↓

▶ Continue CPR, intubate when possible, IV, check ECG rhythm

↓

▶ Epinephrine, 1 mg (1:10,000 solution) IVP every 3–5 minutes (ET dose 2.0–2.5 mg)

(May substitute vasopressin 40 units IV/IO for first or second epinephrine dose)

↓

▶ Atropine, 1 mg IVP every 3–5 minutes up to 3 mg
(ET dose 2–3 mg)

↓

▶ *Consider:*
Treatable causes

↓

▶ Assess quality of resuscitation efforts

↓

▶ Consider termination of efforts following adequate resuscitative efforts if no unusual features

Pulseless Electrical Activity (PEA)

Pulseless electrical activity (PEA) is organized electrical activity (pulseless VT) in the absence of detectable pulses by palpation. The rate may be fast or slow, and the QRS complex may be narrow or wide. Table 5-19 lists the features of PEA.

TABLE 5-19 **Pulseless Electrical Activity**

Rhythm	Variable, depends on the underlying rhythm
Rate	Variable, depends on the underlying rhythm
	Rate that appears on monitor has no corresponding pulse
P wave	Variable, may be present or absent, depends on the underlying rhythm
PR interval	Variable, depends on the underlying rhythm
QRS	Variable, width may be $<$ or $>$ 0.12 sec., depends on the underlying rhythm

(continued)

Common causes	6 Hs and 6 Ts:
	■ Hypovolemia
	■ Hypoxia
	■ Hydrogen ion (acidosis)
	■ Hypokalemia/hyperkalemia
	■ Hypoglycemia
	■ Hypothermia
	■ Tablets/toxins (overdose)
	■ Tamponade (cardiac)
	■ Tension pneumothorax
	■ Thrombosis (coronary)
	■ Thrombosis (pulmonary embolism)
	■ Trauma
Signs and symptoms	■ Loss of consciousness
	■ Irregular breathing that rapidly results in apnea
	■ Profound hypotension with no palpable pulses
	■ Absent heart sounds
Management	PEA Algorithm

PEA Algorithm

▶ Primary ABCD survey, CPR

   ↓

▶ Secondary ABCD survey
Continue effective CPR, intubate when possible, IV, check ECG rhythm

   ↓

▶ *Consider:*
Treatable causes
Epinephrine, 1 mg (1:10,000 solution) IVP every 3–5 minutes
(ET dose 2.0–2.5 mg)
(May substitute vasopressin 40 units IV/IO for first or second epinephrine dose)

   ↓

▶ If ECG rhythm rate < 60/min

↓

▶ Atropine, 1 mg IVP every 3–5 minutes up to 3 mg
(ET dose 2–3 mg)

↓

▶ Continue to evaluate for and treat underlying causes

◆ ◆ ◆ Testing Tips

- Recognize that the presence of a cardiac rhythm does not mean the patient has a pulse! Keep your hand on the femoral pulse at all times to assess the effects of your resuscitation.
- Give atropine only if the rate is slow.

The Bottom Line

The ECG reflects the electrical activity of the heart. It is important to treat an abnormal ECG rhythm within the context of the patient's overall condition. You must assess how the rhythm affects the patient's perfusion status. To do this, perform the following:

- Observe the patient's level of consciousness.
- Assess the patient's skin color, temperature, and moisture.
- Measure the pulse, blood pressure, respiration rate, and oxygen saturation.
- Auscultate the patient's breath and heart sounds.

Once you perform these steps, then you will be prepared to choose the appropriate action to treat the patient—not just the rhythm.

6

Acute Coronary Syndromes

To successfully manage patients who may be presenting with an acute coronary syndrome (ACS), you must have a high index of suspicion. There are many causes of chest pain that may mimic an acute coronary syndrome. Also, some patients who have an ACS will present with atypical complaints. The goal, therefore, is to have a strategy to use when caring for all patients who present with chest pain. This strategy should include the following elements:

- A thorough history and physical exam
- Risk factor identification and stratification
- 12-lead ECG interpretation
- Cardiac enzyme measurements
- The reevaluation of risk related to negative, indeterminate, or nondiagnostic studies
- Proper treatment (see Algorithm for Ischemic Chest Pain), disposition, and follow-up

◆ ◆ ◆ **Testing Tips**

- For the ACLS course, you will discuss how to examine a patient and look at the ECG. The interpretation will be plainly provided to you, but the review in this chapter should help you recognize the hallmarks of the diagnostic ECG.
- ACS is a continuum of syndromes. Reevaluate the patient often to see where he or she falls on the continuum.

Acute Coronary Syndromes

Acute coronary syndromes are cardiac diseases that result when an atheromatous plaque erodes or ruptures. They include:

- Stable angina
  - Blood vessels narrow, and blood flow cannot always meet the needs of the heart.
- Unstable angina
  - Anginal symptoms are new, occur with increasing frequency, and are independent of activity.
- Non-Q-wave MI
  - This type of MI usually involves incomplete coronary occlusion.
  - The clot often dissolves spontaneously.
  - Fibrinolytic therapy may be helpful.
- Q-wave MI
  - This type of MI results in a complete, permanent coronary occlusion.
  - Permanent infarction of some myocardial tissue will result.
  - The area surrounding the infarct area (penumbra) may be saved.

The 12-Lead ECG and Cardiac Anatomy

The 12-lead ECG gives you a view of the heart that will help you:

- Determine if the patient is having ST-segment-elevation myocardial infarction (STEMI)
- Detect ischemic ECG changes
- Assess for conduction delays
- Distinguish among arrhythmias

The 12-lead ECG is just one assessment tool to help you form your clinical impression. Thorough assessment of a 12-lead ECG is a complex art that takes time to master. Many patients who are having an MI will have a normal initial 12-lead ECG, so you should interpret the ECG results within the context of the entire patient assessment. If your initial ECG findings cause you to suspect a right ventricular infarct, you may need to perform a 15-lead ECG to view that side of the heart. Your initial course of action will be guided according to the category you assign the patient based upon your initial interpretation of the 12-lead ECG. These categories are:

- ST-segment-elevation MI (STEMI)
  - ST-segment elevation
  - New or presumed new left bundle branch block (LBBB)
- High-risk unstable angina (UA) or non-ST-segment-elevation MI (NSTEMI)
  - ST-segment depression
  - T-wave inversion

- Intermediate/low-risk UA
  - Normal or nondiagnostic changes on the ECG

This chapter will focus primarily on assessment and management of the patient in the STEMI category. Patients categorized in the other groups will be discussed later in this text.

ST-Segment Assessment

When assessing the ST segment, use the PR segment as the baseline. The normal ST segment returns to the baseline. To detect ST-segment elevation or depression, find the J point (the point that marks the end of the QRS and the beginning of the ST segment). Then move one small box (0.04 seconds) past the J point and measure the distance from the baseline to the ST segment (Figure 6-1).

ST-Segment Elevation

Injury to the myocardium produces ST-segment elevation < 1 mm (0.1 mV) in the leads that view the affected area of the heart (Figure 6-2). When ST-segment elevation is present in two or more contiguous leads in a patient with the signs and symptoms of ACS, it is classified as ST-segment-elevation myocardial infarction (STEMI). This means an area of the heart is hypoxic. If you don't intervene quickly to initiate a reperfusion therapy, permanent death of some heart muscle will likely occur.

ST-Segment Depression

ST-segment depression ≥ 0.5 mm (0.05 mV) in two or more contiguous leads that lasts for 20 minutes or more is a sign of myocardial ischemia (Figure 6-3). If the patient has chest pain or discomfort and ST-segment depression, you will treat them for high-risk unstable angina (UA)/non-ST-segment-elevation MI (NSTEMI).

T-Wave Inversion

T-wave inversion is another sign of myocardial ischemia that, in the presence of signs or symptoms of ACS, is considered evidence of UA or NSTEMI. The leads adjacent to the ischemic area of the heart will reflect this change (Figure 6-4). The ischemic T wave is symmetrical.

Left Bundle Branch Block (LBBB)

Some patients with hypertension or preexisting heart disease have a preexisting left bundle branch block (LBBB). But a patient who presents with signs and symptoms of ACS who has a new, or presumed new, LBBB should be treated as having an acute injury to the myocardium. Ideally, an old ECG should be available for comparison to make this diagnosis. The characteristics of left bundle branch block are:

- QRS > 0.12 sec
- In lead V1 (Figure 6-5):
  - Initial small r wave and deep, wide S wave or
  - Absent r wave and deep, wide QS wave

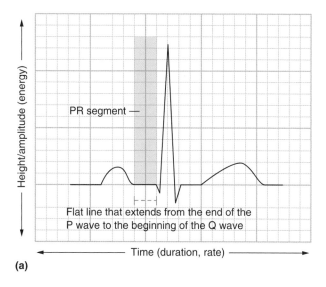

(a)

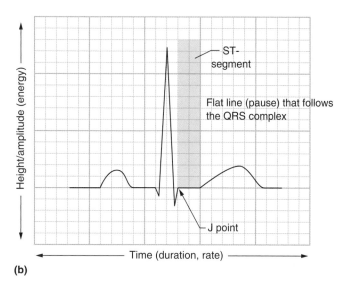

(b)

FIGURE 6-1 Assessing the ST-segment for elevation or depression. (a). The PR-segment can be used as a baseline when evaluating changes in the ST-segment. (b) The ST-segment begins at the J point immediately after the QRS complex. Measure ST-segment elevation one small box (0.04 second) after the J point.

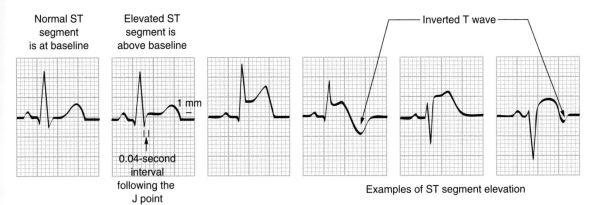

FIGURE 6-2   ST-segment elevation.

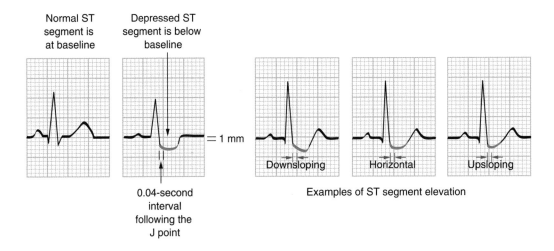

FIGURE 6-3   ST-segment depression.

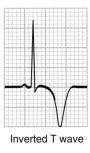

Inverted T wave

FIGURE 6-4   T-wave inversion.

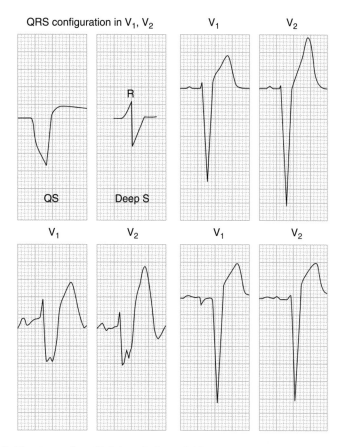

FIGURE 6-5 Examples of left bundle branch block (LBBB) seen in lead V1. Reprinted from *The ECG in Emergency Decision Making,* 2e, by Wellen and Conover, pp. 20 & 21, Copyright 2006, with permission from Elsevier. Reprinted from *Basic Dysrhythmias: Interpretations & Management,* 2e, by Robert J. Huszar, p. 217, Copyright 1994, with permission from Elsevier.

Localizing the Area of Injury or Infarction

When you establish that there is injury or infarction to the heart, you must also determine what area of the heart muscle and what coronary vessels are involved. This will help you follow the appropriate course of action and predict complications.

Table 6-1 provides information on 12-lead ECG changes and cardiac anatomy. Figures 6-6 through 6-11 illustrate the various types of cardiac injury and infarction.

TABLE 6-1 **12-Lead ECG Changes and Cardiac Anatomy**

Ventricle	Injury/Infarct Location	Leads Reflecting ECG Changes	Probable Coronary Artery Affected	ST Segment
Left	Septum	V_1, V_2	LAD, septal branch	Elevation
Left	Anterior	V_3, V_4	LAD, diagonal branch	Elevation
Left	Anteroseptal	V_1, V_2, V_3, V_4	LAD	Elevation
Left	Anterolateral	I, aVL, V_3, V_4, V_5, V_6	LAD, LCX	Elevation
Left	Lateral	I, aVL, V_5, V_6	LCX	Elevation
Left	Inferior	II, III, aVf	RCA	Elevation
Left	Inferolateral	I, II, III, aVL, aVF, V_5, V_6	RCA, LCX	Elevation
Left	Posterior	V_1, V_2, V_3, V_4	LCX or RCA	Depression
Right	Right ventricle	V_4R, V_5R	RCA	Elevation

LAD = left anterior descending (of the coronary artery), LCX = left circumflex branch (of the left coronary artery), RCA = right coronary artery

 Serum Markers Used to Assess ACS

Cardiac biomarkers (enzymes) are substances released from the heart when it is injured. Blood tests that detect increases in these biomarkers help diagnose MI, determine the risk of UA or MI, and predict patient outcome. When the patient has elevated cardiac enzymes, anticipate complications related to myocardial infarction. You may not be able to rely on the markers to assist with your diagnosis in the early care of your patient because the markers will be positive only if the patient has had pain for 6 to 8 hours. Reperfusion treatment should not be delayed to wait on blood marker results if the patient has ECG evidence of STEMI. Blood markers that will be elevated in the presence of injury to the myocardium include:

- Cardiac troponin I or T
- Creatine kinase isoenzyme (CK-MB)

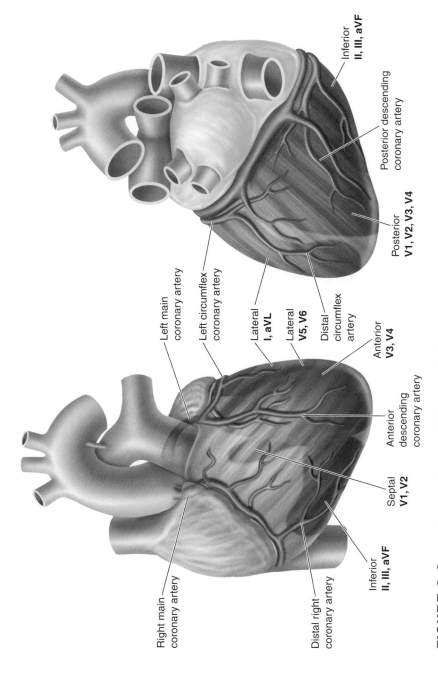

Right main
coronary artery

Left main
coronary artery

Left circumflex
coronary artery

Lateral
I, aVL

Lateral
V5, V6

Distal
circumflex
artery

Distal right
coronary artery

Anterior
descending
coronary artery

Anterior
V3, V4

Septal
V1, V2

Inferior
II, III, aVF

Inferior
II, III, aVF

Posterior descending
coronary artery

Posterior
V1, V2, V3, V4

FIGURE 6-6   Localization of myocardial injury and infarction.

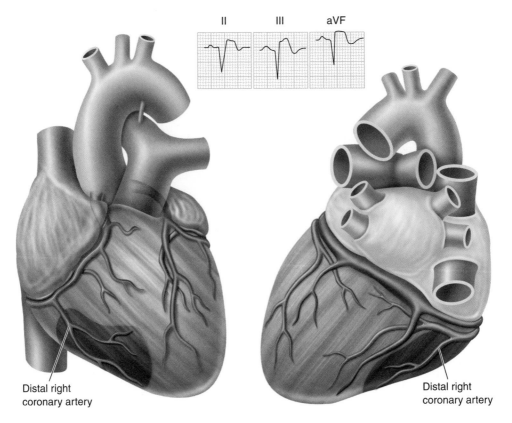

Distal right
coronary artery

Distal right
coronary artery

FIGURE 6-7   Inferior infarction.

Algorithm for Ischemic Chest Pain

▶ Primary ABCD survey

▶ O$_2$; IV; cardiac monitor; assess vital signs; attach pulse oximeter; obtain history, physical exam, 12- or 15-lead ECG promptly, serum cardiac markers, electrolyte and coagulation studies, and portable chest X-ray; have a defibrillator accessible

▶ Immediate general treatment
Oxygen, 4 L/min
Aspirin, 160–325 mg
Nitroglycerin (NTG), sublingual, spray, or IV

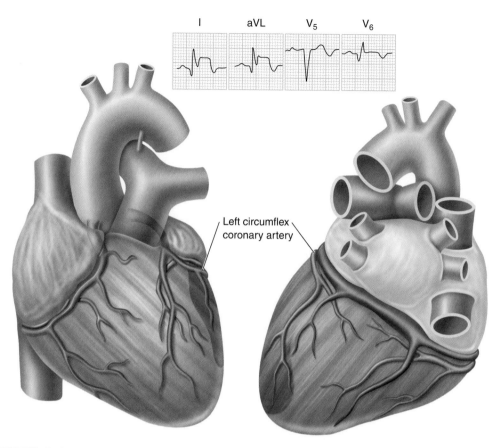

FIGURE 6-8   Lateral infarction.

Morphine IV if pain not relieved with NTG

▶ Evaluate the 12- or 15-lead ECG and classify the patient into one of three categories:
Category 1: ST-segment elevation or new left bundle branch block (LBBB) (ST-segment-elevation MI)
Category 2: ST-segment depression (≥ 0.5 mm) or dynamic T-wave inversion
  ● Non-ST-segment-elevation MI (NSTEMI) if serum cardiac markers reveal troponin is present
  ● Unstable angina if serum cardiac markers are negative
Category 3: A nondiagnostic or normal ECG

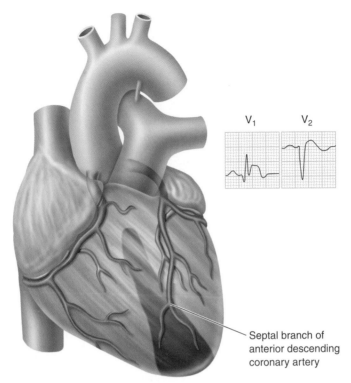

FIGURE 6-9   Septal infarction.

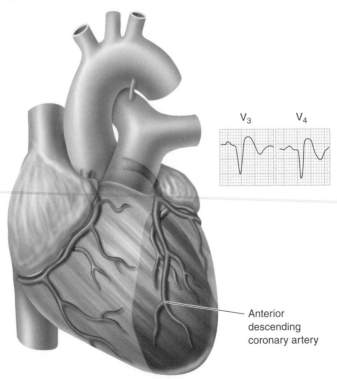

FIGURE 6-10   Anterior infarction.

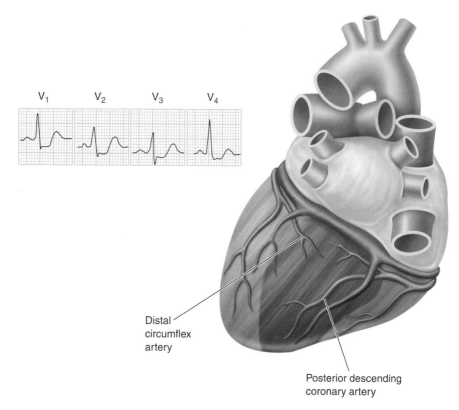

FIGURE 6-11 Posterior infarction. A posterior infarction may result from occlusion of the distal portion of the left circumflex artery or the posterior descending artery, which is formed by the right coronary artery in most patients.

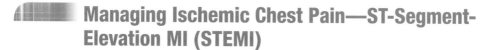

◆ ◆ ◆ **Testing Tips**

- The patient should be placed into one of these three categories within 10 minutes of arrival in the ED so appropriate treatment can begin.

Managing Ischemic Chest Pain—ST-Segment-Elevation MI (STEMI)

The effectiveness of interventions for STEMI is time-dependent. Act quickly to initiate the appropriate reperfusion therapy so circulation can be restored to the coronary arteries and so complications can be prevented.

Treatment Goals for Acute Coronary Syndromes

When caring for patients who present with an ACS, your primary objectives should be to:

- Minimize myocardial necrosis
  - Optimize function of the left ventricle
  - Prevent heart failure
- Prevent adverse cardiac events
  - Death
  - MI
- Manage immediate life-threatening ACS complications, such as arrhythmias

Specific Interventions for STEMI

Treatment measures vary according to patient history, signs and symptoms, and risk factors. Interventions that you should consider when caring for your patient with STEMI include:

- Reperfusion therapy
- Oxygen
- Aspirin or clopidogrel
- Nitrates
- Morphine
- Heparin (if using fibrin-specific fibrinolytics)
- GP IIb/IIIa inhibitors
- Beta-blockers (if not contraindicated)
- Angiotensin-converting enzyme (ACE) inhibitors (after 6 hours or when stable)

Reperfusion Therapy

There are three measures that may be used to restore circulation to an occluded coronary blood vessel:

- Fibrinolytic drugs
- Percutaneous coronary intervention (PCI)
- Surgery to revascularize the coronary arteries

Fibrinolytic Drugs

Fibrinolytic drugs may be used to treat STEMI if fewer than 12 hours have passed since the onset of symptoms. Rapid treatment of STEMI using fibrinolytic drugs is the preferred intervention if:

- Signs and symptoms have been present for < 3 hours.
- There is no contraindication to fibrinolysis.

- Timely access to PCI is not an option.
  - Door to balloon time is > 90 minutes.
  - PCI would be delayed > 1 hour after fibrinolysis could be given.

Fibrinolytic drugs convert plasminogen to plasmin and dissolve blood clots. The chief side effect is severe bleeding. Fibrinolytic drugs used to treat STEMI include:

- Alteplase (Activase; tissue plasminogen activator [tPA])
- Reteplase (Retavase)
- Streptokinase (Streptase)
- Tenecteplase (TNKase)

Fibrinolysis Exclusion Criteria

Carefully assess the patient prior to administering fibrinolytic drugs and weigh the risk of administration against the benefit. Use Table 6-2 as a guideline for clinical decision-making. It may not be all-inclusive or definitive.

Percutaneous Coronary Intervention (PCI)

The most common type of percutaneous coronary intervention (PCI) used to acutely treat STEMI is coronary angioplasty. This procedure is sometimes accompanied by placement of a stent to keep the coronary vessel patent. In hospitals that perform a large number of these procedures in less than 90 minutes from the patient's arrival to the ED, survival using PCI is better than with fibrinolysis.

Revascularization Surgery

Emergency coronary artery bypass graft (CABG) is rarely a first-line intervention for management of acute STEMI. It should be considered if:

- The patient is still symptomatic after unsuccessful PCI and surgery would be helpful.
- The patient is not a candidate for fibrinolysis or PCI and still has ischemic symptoms.
- Repair of a ventricular septal rupture is needed.
- The patient has cardiogenic shock (in selected, very specific cases only).
- There are ventricular arrhythmias in a patient with significant left mainstem occlusion or when there is disease of three coronary blood vessels.

Other Pharmacologic Interventions

There are many drugs that you can give to treat a patient with an ACS. Prior to administering any of these drugs, carefully consider the indications and contraindications relative to your specific patient.

Morphine Sulfate

Morphine sulfate is an opiate analgesic drug given to patients with ACS who are still experiencing pain after administration of nitroglycerin. Morphine reduces anxiety and

TABLE 6-2   **Contraindications and Cautions for Fibrinolysis Use in ST-Segment-Elevation Myocardial Infarction**

Absolute Exclusion Criteria

- Any prior ICH
- Known structural cerebral vascular lesion (e.g., AVM)
- Known malignant intracranial neoplasm (primary or metastatic)
- Ischemic stroke within 3 months *EXCEPT* ischemic stroke within 3 hours
- Suspected aortic dissection
- Active bleeding or bleeding diathesis (excluding menses)
- Significant closed head or facial trauma within 3 months

Relative Contraindications

- History of chronic, severe, poorly controlled hypertension
- Severe uncontrolled hypertension on presentation (SBP greater than 180 mmHg or DBP greater than 110 mmHg)*
- History of prior ischemic stroke greater than 3 months, dementia, or known intracranial pathology not covered in contraindications
- Traumatic or prolonged (> 10 minutes) CPR or major surgery (< 3 weeks)
- Recent internal bleeding (within 2–4 weeks)
- Noncompressible vascular punctures
- For streptokinase/anisreplase, prior exposure (> 5 days prior) or prior allergic reaction to these agents
- Pregnancy
- Active peptic ulcer
- Current use of anticoagulants: the higher the INR, the higher the risk of bleeding

AVM = arteriovenous malformation, DBP = diastolic blood pressure, ICH = intracranial hemorrhage, INR = International Normalized Ratio, SBP = systolic blood pressure

*Could be an absolute contraindication in low-risk patients with ST-segment-elevation myocardial infarction.

Source: Adapted from "ACC/AHA Guidelines for the Management of Patients with ST-Elevation Myocardial Infarction: Executive Summary: A Report of the ACC/AHA Task Force on Practice Guidelines (Committee to Revise the 1999 Guidelines (Committee to Revise the 1999 Guidelines on the Management of Patients with Acute Myocardial Infarction)," by E. M. Antman, et al., *Circulation* 110, pp. 588-636, August 2004.

dilates the patient's arteries and veins. This decreases the cardiac preload and afterload, and therefore reduces the work of the heart.

Oxygen

The AHA recommends oxygen administration in STEMI during the first 6 hours of treatment. Administer oxygen at 4 L/min by nasal cannula. If the patient's oxygen saturation drops below 90% or pulmonary congestion develops, increase the oxygen delivery.

Nitroglycerin

Nitroglycerin is given to relieve the pain associated with ACS. It causes arterial and venous dilation, including of the coronary arteries. This dilation lowers cardiac preload and afterload, decreasing the work of the heart. You may give up to 3 doses of sublingual nitroglycerin to relieve pain associated with ACS. IV nitroglycerin is indicated for patients who are hypertensive, have unrelieved chest pain, or have pulmonary congestion.

If your patient has an inferior MI with right ventricular (RV) involvement, use nitroglycerin with *extreme* caution, if at all (consult with local experts). The administration of nitroglycerin in these patients may cause profound hypotension. If that occurs, place the patient in the modified Trendelenburg position and administer a fluid bolus.

Do not use nitroglycerin if the patient has:

- SBP < 90 mmHg (or 30 mmHg below the normal baseline)
- HR < 50 bpm
- HR > 100 bpm
- Taken a phosphodiesterase inhibitor for erectile dysfunction within 24 hours (within 48 hours for tadalafil [Cialis])

Aspirin

It is important that you administer aspirin early if you suspect ACS. Aspirin has antiplatelet effects. This action decreases further clot extension and helps to prevent clots from developing again after reperfusion therapy. Non-enteric, chewable aspirin is preferred because it is absorbed more quickly. You may administer aspirin by rectal suppository if the patient is vomiting.

Clopidogrel

Clopidogrel inhibits platelet aggregation by a different mechanism than aspirin. It is given:

- As an alternative to aspirin in patients with a known aspirin allergy
- With aspirin to patients who will undergo PCI with stent insertion

Heparin

Heparin interferes with blood coagulation by indirectly inhibiting thrombin. It prevents the formation of new clots and the extension of existing ones; however, heparin does not dissolve existing clots. Heparin is used as an adjunct to aspirin and other platelet inhibitors in the treatment of STEMI or UA. The dose of heparin varies according to the specific fibrinolytic drug it is given with. Prior to giving heparin, screen patients carefully for bleeding risk.

Unfractionated Heparin (UFH)

Give your patient unfractionated heparin if:

- You will be giving them alteplase, reteplase, or tenecteplase.
- They will be having PCI or CABG.

- They are going to be treated with streptokinase, anistreplase, or urokinase and their risk for emboli is high, as in
  - Large or anterior MI
  - Atrial fibrillation
  - History of embolus
  - Left ventricular (LV) thrombus

Low-Molecular-Weight Heparin (LMWH)

LMWH, such as enoxaparin, is sometimes used as an alternative to UHF when given with fibrinolytic therapy if the patient is less than 75 years old and has normal renal function.

Glycoprotein IIb/IIIa Receptor Inhibitors

Glycoprotein (GP) IIb/IIIa receptor inhibitors prevent platelet aggregation by inhibiting the binding of fibrinogen to the glycoprotein IIb/IIIa receptor sites on platelets. You should give GP IIb/IIIa receptor inhibitors as soon as possible before PCA in patients with STEMI. Glyoprotein IIb/III a inhibitors include:

- Abciximab (Reopro)
- Eptifibatide (Integrilin)
- Tirofiban (Aggrastat)

Beta-Blockers

Beta-blockers block sympathetic stimulation of the heart. This slows the heart rate and decreases myocardial contractility. Treating your patient with a beta-blocker reduces myocardial oxygen use and can lower the risk of ventricular arrhythmias after STEMI. The appropriate use of beta-blockers is associated with a significant improvement in long-term survival.[1] Consider administering beta-blockers in all patients with STEMI if no contraindications are present. After administration, monitor the patient for congestive heart failure, shock, and AV block. Beta-blocker drugs that are administered to STEMI patients include:

- Atenolol
- Esmolol
- Labetolol
- Metoprolol
- Propranolol

Angiotensin-Converting Enzyme (ACE) Inhibitors

The early oral administration of ACE inhibitors improves survival and decreases the incidence of congestive heart failure after an MI.[1] You should definitely consider administering ACE inhibitors in patients with STEMI who have:

- Pulmonary congestion
- LV ejection fraction $< 40\%$ (if SBP > 100 mmHg)
- No contraindications to the use of ACE inhibitors
- Heart failure in MI caused by systolic dysfunction

ACE inhibitor drugs used to treat patients with ACS include:

- Captopril
- Enalapril
- Lisinopril
- Ramipril

Complications Related to STEMI

Continually assess and monitor your patient for life-threatening complications that may occur as a result of STEMI. These include:

- Arrhythmias
- Congestive heart failure
- Myocardial rupture

Arrhythmias

The risk of ventricular fibrillation is greatest in the first 4 hours after the onset of symptoms in STEMI. The AHA recommends the following treatment guidelines to prevent or manage ventricular arrhythmias associated with STEMI:[2]

- Do not routinely give lidocaine to prevent ventricular fibrillation after STEMI.
- Do not treat premature ventricular contractions (PVCs) or nonsustained ventricular tachycardia unless they are causing hemodynamic compromise.
- Administer IV beta-blockers if not contraindicated.
- Monitor serum potassium and magnesium levels and maintain them within normal limits.
- Ensure that a defibrillator and appropriate resuscitation equipment are readily available.

---

[1]Ibid.
[2]America Heart Association, "AHA Guidelines for Cardiopulmonary Resuscitation and Emergency Cardiovascular Care," *Circulation* 112, suppl. 1 (2005).

Anticipate bradycardia or heart block development when you are caring for a patient with an acute inferior STEMI. If a symptomatic bradycardia develops, apply the pacing pads and prepare to pace unless other treatments rapidly stabilize your patient.

Congestive Heart Failure

Anticipate congestive heart failure if your patient has a large anterior STEMI. The use of nitrates and morphine are particularly helpful in patients with infarcts that affect the anterior left ventricle. Administer fluids very cautiously in these patients to avoid congestive heart failure from fluid overload. Monitor breath sounds often. Crackles (rales) signal the onset of congestive heart failure.

Myocardial Rupture

Cardiac rupture is a possible complication after STEMI. Patients who have an increased risk for this complication include those with:

- Small first infarcts
- Hypertension and left ventricular hypertrophy
- Lateral MI

Signs and symptoms associated with myocardial rupture vary according to the area of the heart affected. Myocardial rupture may occur in the following are three areas:

- Ventricular septum
- Ventricular free wall
- Papillary muscle

Start beta-blocker treatment early to reduce the risk of this complication. The incidence of some types of myocardial rupture decreases with early reperfusion treatment.

The Team Approach to Clinical Decision-Making in STEMI

Each of the interventions to reduce morbidity and mortality after STEMI is time-sensitive. To be most effective, you must initiate them as quickly as possible. To ensure that each step of the process is performed promptly, everyone involved in the myocardial care continuum must take the right actions at the right time and get the patient to the right care area. The key initial participants in this continuum of care are the patient, the prehospital providers, and the ED staff.

Patient Role

To begin the sequence of prompt emergency cardiac care, the patient has two responsibilities:

1. Recognize that they have signs and symptoms that suggest an ACS
2. Seek appropriate care immediately (call 911 or the local emergency access number)

Prehospital Role

More than 50% of the patients who die after an MI arrest in the prehospital setting. To effectively manage these emergencies and reduce death from sudden cardiac arrest, communities must adopt programs geared to provide the following:

- Early recognition of the symptoms of ACS
- Rapid access to the EMS system
  - Dispatchers may also be trained to tell patients with ACS to take aspirin prior to EMS arrival.
- Early CPR
- Early access to an AED or defibrillator
- Early advanced cardiac care

Advanced EMS providers should ideally:

- Administer oxygen, aspirin, nitroglycerin, and morphine.
- Acquire, interpret, and transmit 12-lead ECGs.
- Screen patients to determine if they are candidates for fibrinolysis.
- Transport patients to appropriate hospitals.
  - A hospital with interventional therapy is needed:
    - With cardiogenic shock
    - With pulmonary edema
    - With a large infarction
    - When fibrinolytics are contraindicated

In some specific, controlled prehospital settings, fibrinolytic therapy may be initiated. This therapy is ideal for symptoms that last 30 minutes to 6 hours. Fibrinolytic therapy requires an organized system with rigorous training and oversight. Consider initiating fibrinolytic therapy if appropriate screening is available.

Emergency Department Role

The emergency department (ED) should establish an organized process to quickly receive, assess, and appropriately treat the patient with ACS. Specific goals an ED should try to achieve include:

- Within 10 minutes:
  - History and physical assessment
  - 12-lead ECG
  - Determination of the appropriate patient category and treatment path
- Within 30 minutes:
  - Fibrinolytic therapy if indicated

- Within 90 minutes:
  - PCI if indicated

◇ ◇ ◇ Testing Tips

- Perform your initial assessment, including a 12-lead ECG, within 10 minutes.
- Notify the appropriate healthcare team members immediately if you identify ST elevation on the 12-lead ECG.
- Don't forget to give chewable aspirin early to the patient with chest pain.

The Bottom Line

Advances in the care of patients with ACS have been revolutionary in the past 15 years. But effectively employing treatments to prevent complications and death from acute coronary syndromes requires a team approach. To try to minimize damage to the heart and lower the risk of life-threatening complications, each member of the team must do the following four things:

1. Quickly recognize that their patient has an ACS.
2. Categorize the patient after interpreting the patient's 12-lead ECG.
3. Select an appropriate treatment path.
4. Rapidly initiate care and diagnostics.

7

Acute Ischemic Stroke

Stroke is the third leading cause of death in this country. Recognition and management of the patient suffering a stroke is as time-sensitive and potentially life-threatening as ACS and other emergency cardiac conditions. If you use a rapid, systematic approach when you care for stroke patients, you can optimize your patients' chance for a good outcome.

Defining Stroke

Stroke occurs when a sudden interruption of cerebral blood flow produces neurologic signs and symptoms. The resulting damage—and the patient's signs and symptoms—depends on the magnitude of the interruption, the area of the brain that is involved, and the effectiveness of collateral blood flow to the affected area of brain.

The two main pipelines that supply blood to the brain are the following:

- Anterior circulation
  - Arises from the carotid arteries
  - Supplies blood to 80% of the brain
- Posterior circulation
  - Supplied by the vertebral arteries
  - Supplies the cerebellum and brainstem

Types of Stroke

Stroke is divided into two main categories: ischemic stroke and hemorrhagic stroke.

Ischemic Stroke

More than 80% of strokes are ischemic strokes (Figure 7-1). There are several types of ischemic strokes:

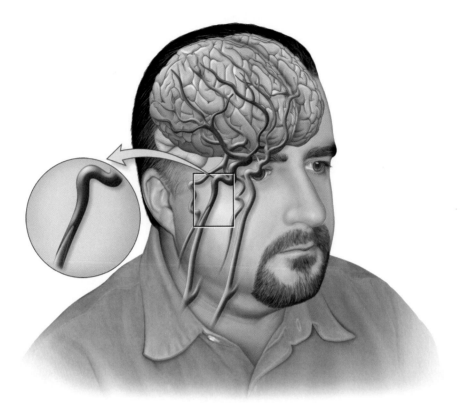

FIGURE 7-1   Ischemic stroke. An ischemic stroke occurs when a blood vessel that supplies blood to the brain becomes blocked, impairing blood flow to part of the brain.

- Thrombotic strokes
  - Develop from ulcerated atherosclerotic plaques
- Small-vessel strokes
  - Result when small emboli block cerebral blood vessels
  - Common in hypertensive patients
- Cardioembolic strokes
  - Develop from a clot that travels from the heart and interrupts blood flow to the brain
  - Most are secondary to atrial fibrillation

Hemorrhagic Stroke

Hemorrhagic stroke occurs when a blood vessel that supplies the brain ruptures and begins to bleed (Figure 7-2). Bleeding from hemorrhagic strokes may be found within the brain tissue (intracerebral) or between the meninges that cover the brain (subarachnoid hemorrhage [SAH]). Causes of hemorrhagic stroke include:

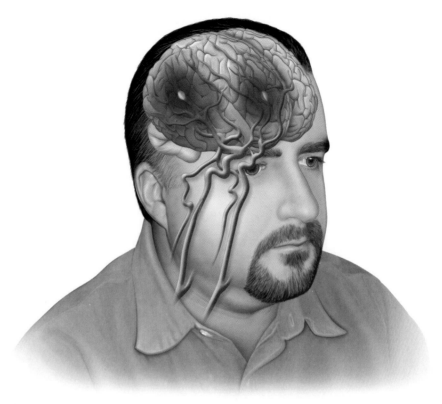

FIGURE 7-2   Hemorrhagic stroke. A hemorrhagic stroke occurs when a weakened blood vessel that supplies blood to the brain ruptures and bleeds.

- Spontaneous intracranial hemorrhage
  - Hypertension is a major risk factor.
- Drug use that causes a rapid increase in blood pressure
- Anticoagulant use
- Tumors
- Arteriovenous malformations (AVMs)
- Aneurysms

 ## Transient Ischemic Attack (TIA)

Transient ischemic attacks have a presentation similar to that of stroke, but the symptoms resolve within 24 hours (many resolve within 30 minutes). Patients who experience a TIA have a very high risk of having a stroke.

Clinical Presentation of Stroke

The signs and symptoms of stroke vary according to the area of the brain affected and the type of stroke (Figure 7-3). Table 7-1 summarizes some of the clinical features you may see during stroke.

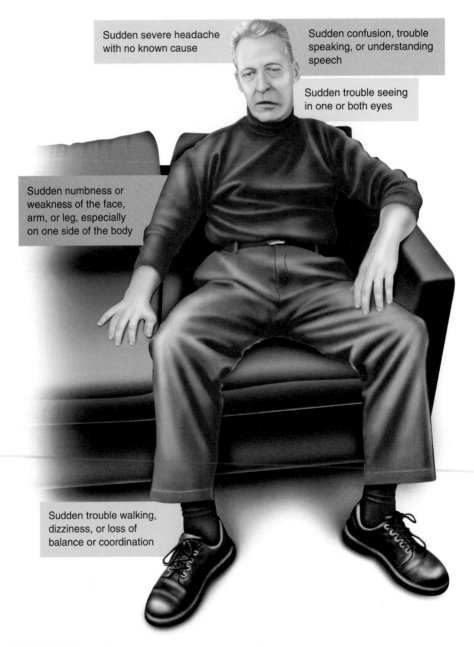

Sudden severe headache with no known cause

Sudden confusion, trouble speaking, or understanding speech

Sudden trouble seeing in one or both eyes

Sudden numbness or weakness of the face, arm, or leg, especially on one side of the body

Sudden trouble walking, dizziness, or loss of balance or coordination

FIGURE 7-3 The signs and symptoms of stroke.

TABLE 7-1 Clinical Features of Stroke

	Ischemic Stroke, Anterior	Ischemic Stroke, Posterior	Hemorrhagic Stroke
Onset	May occur suddenly or have stuttering onset	Varies from minutes (more common) to days or weeks	Sudden onset
Symptom progression	20% of patients get worse within the first 24 hours	40% of patients get worse within the first 3 days	Focal deficits progress over minutes
Mental status	Complete loss of consciousness is rare; may have altered mentation, judgment, and insight	Can present with loss of consciousness, vertigo	Initially, the patient may be agitated or lethargic with progression to unconsciousness; initial transient loss of consciousness suggests SAH
Headache	May be present	May be present	Sudden severe headache: "Worst I've ever had." Aggravated by noise, light.
Sensory	Unilateral hyperesthesia, numbness or loss of sensation in extremities or face	Unilateral or bilateral numbness or tingling of the extremities or face	Sensory deficits on the side of the body opposite the bleeding (less likely with SAH)
Visual/eyes	Blindness in one eye (hemianopsia)	Inability to see well to one side; diplopia (double vision); dysconjugate gaze; inability to recognize visual objects	Pupil response based on the area of the brain affected; may be pinpoint, dilated, unilateral dilated pupil, or sluggish pupil response; papilledema possible
Speech	Aphasia (expressive, receptive, or both)	Dysarthria	
Motor	Paralysis or paresis in extremities on the side opposite brain ischemia	Unilateral or bilateral paralysis or weakness, clumsiness, ataxia	Motor deficits on the side of the body opposite the bleeding
Gastrointestinal	Incontinence may occur	Nausea and vomiting, dysphagia	Nausea and vomiting can be severe

(continued)

Other features	Signs appear on one side of the body only; inattention to one side of the environment	Some signs appear on one side of the face and the opposite side of the body	Markedly elevated blood pressure; symptoms may begin with activity (intercourse, bowel movement, etc.); respiratory pattern may be irregular or deteriorate quickly, needing advanced airway management; stiff neck (SAH)

Stroke Chain of Survival and Recovery

The key actions that must occur to optimize the care and recovery of the patient with stroke have been described by the American Heart Association in their 2005 guidelines:[1]

Detection—Early recognition

Dispatch—Early EMS activation

Delivery—Transport and management

Door—Emergency department triage

Data—Emergency department evaluation and management

Decision—Specific therapies

Drug—Fibrinolytic drug administration

Detection—Recognition of Stroke

The patient often causes the first delay in stroke recognition and care. This is usually related to:

- Failure to recognize the signs and symptoms of stroke
- A lack of understanding that urgent care is needed

Dispatch

Even when the patient or family recognizes that the signs and symptoms indicate a stroke, they may delay seeking care. Community education programs should urge patients who think they are having a stroke to do the following:

- Call 911 and go to the hospital by ambulance immediately
- Not delay care by calling someone else (physician, family) before seeking care

---

[1]American Heart Association, "AHA Guidelines for Cardiopulmonary Resuscitation and Emergency Cardiovascular Care," *Circulation* 112, suppl. 1 (2005): IV-111-120.

Delivery—Prehospital Assessment and Management

To provide optimal care to the stroke patient, prehospital providers should:

- Perform a rapid initial assessment.
- Protect and maintain the airway.
- Apply oxygen if the patient's SaO_2 is <92%.
- Assist ventilation if needed.
- Initiate an IV en route to the hospital.
- Monitor the ECG and treat symptomatic rhythm disturbances.
- Monitor vital signs.
- Assess blood glucose and treat hypoglycemia if it is present.
- Use consistent assessment tools to rapidly assess stroke.
- Determine the time of onset of stroke symptoms.
- Provide rapid transport to a hospital with appropriate resources to care for the stroke patient.

Use the Cincinnati Prehospital Stroke Scale and/or the Los Angeles Prehospital Stroke Screen to quickly assess for the presence of signs and symptoms consistent with a stroke. Use the Glasgow Coma Scale to determine the degree of neurological disability. Memorize them or keep them readily available when caring for a potential stroke victim.

Cincinnati Prehospital Stroke Scale

The Cincinnati Prehospital Stroke Scale identifies factors in stroke assessment. See Figure 7-4.

Los Angeles Prehospital Stroke Screen

The Los Angeles Prehospital Stroke Screen (LAPSS) identifies factors in stroke assessment (Table 7-2). It is used for the evaluation of acute, noncomatose, nontraumatic neurologic complaints. If items 1 though 6 are all checked "Yes" (or "Unknown"), provide the hospital with a prearrival notification about the potential stroke patient. If any item is checked "No," return to the appropriate treatment protocol.

In patients who are having a stroke, the LAPSS score will be positive 93% of the time. When the patient has a positive LAPSS score, the chance of stroke is 97%.[2]

Glasgow Coma Scale

Use the Glasgow Coma Scale to assess the degree of neurologic disability (Table 7-3). Reassess the patient's neurologic status often to detect changes in his or her condition.

---

[2]C. S. Kidwell, S. Starkman, M. Eckstein, K. Weems, and J. L. Saver, "Identifying Stroke in the Field: Prospective Validation of the Los Angeles Prehospital Stroke Screen (LAPSS)" *Stroke* 31, no. 1 (Jan. 2000): 71–76. PMID: 10625718.

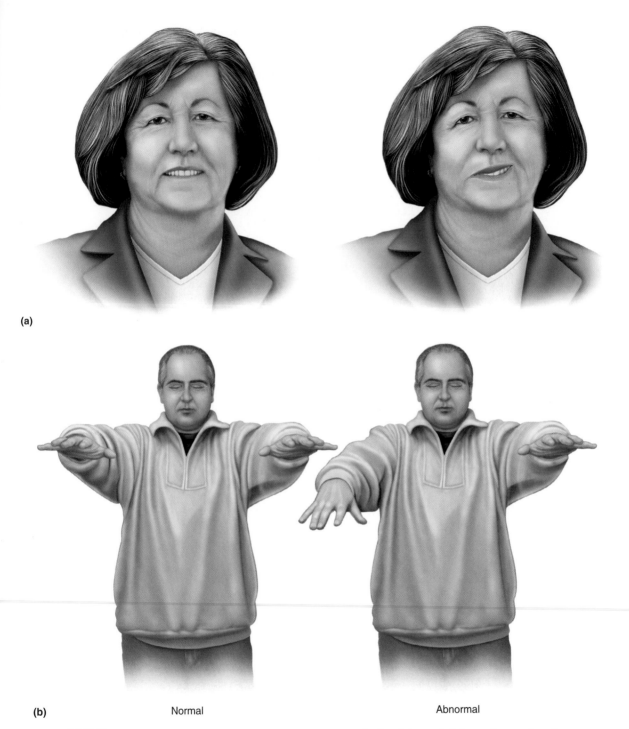

Normal   Abnormal

FIGURE 7-4   Cincinnati Prehospital Stroke Scale. (a) Assess for facial droop. Ask the patient to show her teeth or smile. Normal: Both sides of the face move equally. Abnormal: One side of the face does not move as well as the other side. (b) Assess for arm drift. Have the patient close his eyes and hold both arms straight out for 10 seconds. Normal: The patient is able to move both arms equally, or both arms do not move at all. Abnormal: One arm does not move or one arm drifts down relative to the other.

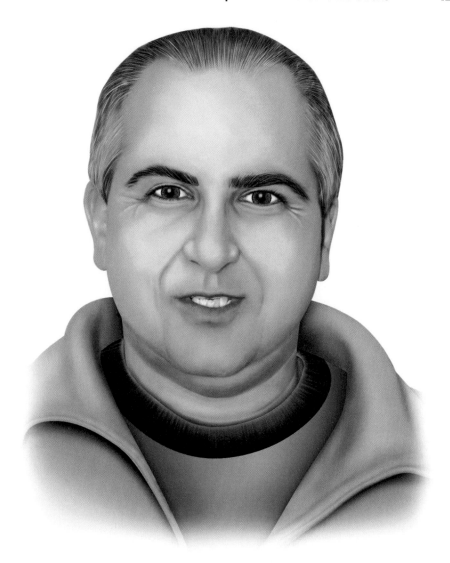

(c)

FIGURE 7-4 *(Continued)*
(c) Assess speech. Ask the patient to say, "The sky is blue over Cincinnati." or "You can't teach an old dog new tricks." Normal: The patient uses the correct words without slurring. Abnormal: The patient slurs his words, uses inappropriate words, or is unable to speak.

Door—Emergency Department Triage of the Stroke Patient

After you determine that the patient is having a stroke, make every attempt to meet the time targets identified by the National Institute of Neurological Disorders and Stroke (NINDS), listed in Table 7-4. When you meet these targets, the patient has the best opportunity for a favorable outcome.

TABLE 7-2   Los Angeles Prehospital Stroke Screen (LAPSS)

Screening Criteria*	Yes	Unknown	No
1. Age over 45 years	_____	_____	_____
2. No prior history of seizure disorder	_____	_____	_____
3. New onset of neurologic symptoms in last 24 hours	_____	_____	_____
4. Patient was ambulatory at baseline (prior to event)	_____	_____	_____
5. Blood glucose between 60 and 400 mg/dL	_____	_____	_____

Exam: Look for obvious asymmetry	Normal	Right	Left
Facial smile/ grimace	_____	_____ Droop	_____ Droop
Grip	_____	_____ Weak grip	_____ Weak grip
		_____ No grip	_____ No grip
Arm weakness	_____	_____ Drifts down	_____ Drifts down
		_____ Falls rapidly	_____ Falls rapidly

	Yes	No
6. Based on exam, patient has only unilateral weakness.	_____	_____

* If yes (or unknown) to all items above, LAPSS screening criteria have been met. If LAPSS criteria for stroke are met, call the receiving hospital with "code stroke." If not, return to the appropriate treatment protocol. (**Note:** The patient may still be experiencing a stroke, even if LAPSS criteria are not met.)

Source: Adapted with permission from C. S. Kidwell, S. Starkman, M. Eckstein, K. Weems, and J. L. Saver, "Identifying Stroke in the Field: Prospective Validation of the Los Angeles Prehospital Stroke Screen (LAPSS)" *Stroke* 31, no. 1, pp. 71-76, January 2000. Copyright Lippincott, Williams & Wilkins. (http://ww.com)

Door—Emergency Department Care of the Stroke Patient

The ED staff must rapidly assess the stroke patient and determine what interventions are appropriate. Goals of initial ED care include:

- Performing an initial assessment (or repeating it if the patient arrives by ambulance)
  - Managing life threats
- Repeating the Glasgow Coma Scale
- Identifying stroke and differentiating it from conditions with similar presentations
- Determining if the stroke is
  - Hemorrhagic
  - Ischemic

TABLE 7-3 Glasgow Coma Scale

	Response	Score
Eyes open	Spontaneous	4
	To speech	3
	To pain	2
	Absent	1
Verbal response	Converses/oriented	5
	Converses/disoriented	4
	Inappropriate	3
	Incomprehensible	2
	Absent	1
Motor response	Obeys	6
	Localizes pain	5
	Withdraws (flexion)	4
	Abnormal flexion (decorticate)	3
	Abnormal extension (decerebrate)	2
	Absent	1
	Score: E + V + M	15

Source: "Instructions for Scoring the Glasgow Coma Scale from the Head Trauma Research Project," New York University Medical Center, Institute of Rehabilitation Medicine, available at www.biact.org/infractl/flasgow.html.

TABLE 7-4 NINDS-Recommended Stroke Evaluation: Targets for Potential Thrombolytic Candidates.

Activity	Target
Door to physician evaluation	10 minutes
Door to access to neurological expertise (in person or by phone)	15 minutes
Door to computed tomography (CT) scan completion	25 minutes
Door to CT scan interpretation	45 minutes
Door to drug /intervention	60 minutes
Door to neurosurgical availability (on-site or by transport)	2 hours
Door to monitored bed	3 hours

Source: Proceedings of a National Symposium on Rapid Identification and Treatment of Acute Stroke, December 12–13, 1996. NINDS: Stroke Proceedings: Bock, www.ninds.nih.gov/news_and_events/proceedings/stroke_proceedings/bock.htm (accessed 8/24/06).

- Completing appropriate diagnostic tests if indicated, including:
  - CT scan
  - Laboratory tests
  - Lumbar puncture (for SAH)
  - Cerebral angiography

Hunt and Hess Scale

If the patient's CT scan indicates a subarachnoid hemorrhage, use the Hunt and Hess Scale to grade its severity and predict survival (Table 7-5). This scale is helpful for communicating the patient's condition to the neurosurgeon.

TABLE 7-5   **Hunt and Hess Scale**

Description of Neurologic Status	Grade	Survival*
Asymptomatic	1	70
Severe headache or nuchal rigidity; no neurologic deficit	2	60
Drowsiness; minimal neurologic deficit	3	50
Stupor; moderate to severe hemiparesis	4	40
Deep coma; decerebrate posturing	5	10

*Predicted 2-month survival (%)

Source: Borrowed with permission from "Stroke," in *Rosen's Emergency Medicine: Concepts and Clinical Practice,* 5th ed., ed.-in-chief J. A. Marx (Mosby, 2002).

Conditions That Mimic Thromboembolic Stroke

There are many illnesses whose signs and symptoms mimic thromboembolic stroke. They include the following:

- Stroke due to vascular dissection
- Stroke due to vasculitis
- Meningitis
- Infectious endocarditis
- Focal neurologic manifestations of psychiatric origin
- Multiple sclerosis
- Migraine
- Venous thrombosis
- Herpes simplex encephalitis
- Status epilepticus
- Neoplasm
- Trauma

- Transient neurologic symptoms due to hypo- or hyperglycemia
- Drug abuse (e.g., cocaine)

Diagnostic Tests to Evaluate Stroke (Data)

The most common imaging study used to diagnose ischemic stroke is the noncontrast CT scan. Significant clinical findings to look for on the CT scan are:

- Blood
  - Indicates a hemorrhagic stroke
  - Indicates the patient is not a candidate for fibrinolytics
- Hypodense areas
  - Results from swelling in the brain after stroke
  - Usually appears no earlier than 3 hours after the stroke
  - Indicates that the patient is not a candidate for fibrinolytics
- Normal findings
  - In the first few hours after an ischemic stroke, the CT scan will be normal.

Other diagnostic tests that may be indicated based on the initial assessment of the patient are:

- Lumbar puncture
  - Perform if the CT is normal but the clinical picture suggests SAH
- Cerebral angiography
  - Perform for SAH with aneurysm

Blood Tests

Obtain the following laboratory tests early in the care of the stroke patient:

- Complete blood count (CBC)
- Platelet count
- International normalized ratio (INR)
- PT/aPTT (prothrombin time/activated partial thromboplastin time)
- Type and screen
- Blood chemistry
  - Electrolytes
  - Blood glucose
    - Treat if hypoglycemic or if blood glucose > 200 mg/dL
- Toxicology screen
  - If toxic exposure is suspected

Fibrinolytic Therapy for Stroke (Decision)

As soon as you begin to suspect that the patient is having an ischemic stroke, start to complete the fibrinolytic checklist for stroke (Table 7-6).

TABLE 7-6   Fibrinolytic Therapy Checklist for Acute Ischemic Stroke

Inclusion Criteria **(All "Yes" boxes must be checked before treatment)**

Yes

> 18 years of age?

Clinical diagnosis of ischemic stroke causing a measurable neurological deficit?

Did the symptoms clearly begin < 3 hours before fibrinolytic treatment would begin?

Exclusion Criteria **(All "No" boxes must be checked before treatment)**

Contraindications

Evidence of intracranial hemorrhage on pretreatment noncontrast head CT?

Uncontrolled hypertension: At the time treatment should begin, SBP > 185 mmHg or DBP > 110 mmHg, when measured more than once

Known arteriovenous malformation, neoplasm, or aneurysm?

Witnessed seizure at stroke onset?

Active internal bleeding or acute trauma (fracture)?

Acute bleeding diathesis, including but not limited to:

- Platelet count < 100,000/mm³?
- Heparin received within 48 hours, resulting in an aPTT that is greater than upper limit of normal for laboratory?
- Current use of anticoagulant (e.g., warfarin sodium) or PT > 15 seconds?*

Within 3 months of intracranial or intraspinal surgery, serious head trauma, or previous stroke?

Arterial puncture at noncompressible site within past 7 days?

* In patients without recurrent use of oral anticoagulants or heparin, treatment with tissue plasminogen activator (tPA) can be initiated before coagulation study results are available but should be discontinued if the INR is > 1.7 or the activated partial thromboplastin time is elevated by local laboratory standards.

Source: Adapted from the *Handbook of Emergency Cardiovascular Care for Healthcare Providers*, p. 20, 2005, the American Cancer Society.

Relative Contraindications and Precautions

Under some circumstances and after carefully weighing the risk-to-benefit ratio, patients may be given fibrinolytic therapy even with one or more relative contraindications. Consider these risks carefully before your team makes the decision to give fibrinolytic treatment:[3]

- Only minor or rapidly improving stroke symptoms (clearing spontaneously)
- Within 14 days of major surgery or serious trauma

[3]Adapted with permission from American Heart Association, *Guidelines Handbook* (2005), p. 20.

- Recent gastrointestinal or urinary tract hemorrhage (within previous 21 days)
- Recent acute MI (within previous 3 months)
- Post–myocardial infarction pericarditis
- Abnormal blood glucose level ($<$ 50 or $>$ 400 mg/dL)

Signs and Symptoms That Suggest Intracranial Hemorrhage Following tPA

You must continually observe the patient for signs and symptoms of intracranial hemorrhage during and after tPA administration. Assess for:

- Increased neurologic deficit, including a deteriorating level of consciousness
- New headache or increasing headache
- Acute hypertension (SBP $>$ 185 mmHg or DBP $>$ 100 mmHg in two successive readings over 10 minutes after infusion of tPA)
- Nausea and vomiting
- Lethargy

Algorithm for the General Management of a Suspected Stroke

Prehospital Care

▶ ABCD survey

↓

▶ Initial assessment, including:
Glasgow Coma Scale
  Cincinnati Prehospital Stroke Scale
  and/or
  Los Angeles Prehospital Stroke Screen

↓

▶ Establish the time patient was last seen *without* symptoms

↓

▶ Immediate transport to the ED (preferably a stroke center); while en route: Notify the hospital:
  - The patient is a "stroke alert" and inform them of the time of symptom onset
  - Glasgow Coma Scale
  - Results of Cincinnati Prehospital Stroke Scale or Los Angeles Prehospital Stroke Screen (positive or negative)
  - If the patient is unstable (e.g., seizures, head trauma, bleeding)
  - If the patient has uncontrolled hypertension

(continued)

- If the patient is taking anticoagulants
O$_2$ to maintain SaO$_2$ > 92%
IV normal saline TKO
Monitor (12-lead ECG, if time permits)
Reassess vital signs often
Check blood glucose level (give 50% dextrose if hypoglycemic)
Treat complications of stroke according to local protocol

Emergency Department

▶ Within 10 minutes of arrival:
- ABCs, O$_2$, IV (if none established), cardiac monitor, vital signs (including pulse oximetry), 12-lead ECG
- Check blood glucose level immediately (if not already done)
  - Give 50% dextrose if hypoglycemic; give insulin if > 200 mg/dL
- Order and obtain lab work, including CBC, electrolytes, clotting studies, comprehensive metabolic panel, and chemistry and lipid profiles
- Order noncontrast CT scan
- Perform general neurologic screening assessment
- Alert stroke team

▶ Within 25 minutes of arrival:
- Review patient history
- Confirm the time of onset of stroke symptoms
- Perform physical and neurologic exam
  - Consider conditions that mimic stroke
  - Confirm that stroke is suspected
- Complete noncontrast CT scan
- Obtain lateral cervical spine X-ray if patient is comatose and trauma is possibly involved

▶ Within 45 minutes of arrival:
- Have CT scan interpreted
- Obtain patient weight

▶ If CT scan shows no intracerebral or subarachnoid hemorrhage:
- Physician or stroke team to determine tPA eligibility
- Determine the following:
- Are any exclusions for tPA present?
- Are neurologic deficits variable or rapidly improving?
- Does the patient still meet the inclusion criteria?

▶ Is the patient still a candidate for fibrinolytic therapy?
- No
  - Give aspirin (if not contraindicated)
  - Provide supportive therapy
  - Consider admission
  - Consider alternative diagnoses and conditions needing treatment
- Yes
  - Discuss fibrinolytic treatment risks/benefits with the patient and family. If acceptable, begin fibrinolytic treatment.
    - tPA dose: 0.9 mg/kg (90-mg max dose)
      - 10% of total dose given IV bolus over 1 minute
      - Give remaining 90% of total dose by continuous IV infusion over 1 hour
  - Monitor neurologic status—STAT CT scan if deterioration
  - Monitor BP, treat as indicated
    - Use arm without the tPA infusion
    - Monitor BP every 15 minutes for 2 hours, then every 30 minutes for 6 hours, and then every hour for 18 hours
  - Admit to critical care unit
  - Do not administer heparin, warfarin, aspirin, Ticlopidine, or other anti-platelet agents for 24 hours
  - Minimize invasive procedures for 24 hours
  - Avoid indwelling bladder catheters if possible
  - Avoid nasogastric tube for first 24 hours after treatment

◆ ◆ ◆ Testing Tips

- Perform a thorough ABCD exam, paying particular attention to the patient's airway.
- Use the stroke scales.
- Determine the time of stroke onset to start the clock for possible thrombolytics.
- If the patient awoke with the stroke symptoms, assume that the onset was the last time the patient was awake and without symptoms.
- Check the blood glucose level.
- Check the 12-lead ECG for possible ischemia or a-fib (atrial fibrillation) or flutter.
- Assess the CT scan results quickly to detect the presence of blood.
- Assess the patient for exclusion criteria for fibrinolytics.

Complications of Stroke

Stroke complications vary according to the location, severity, and type of stroke. Monitor the patient carefully for the following life-threatening conditions that may complicate or accompany stroke.

Airway and Breathing Problems

The patient may have difficulty in maintaining his or her airway because of a decreased level of consciousness, difficulty in swallowing (dysphagia), or vomiting caused by the stroke. Irregular breathing patterns may be present after hemorrhagic stroke. To care for the stroke patient who has airway or breathing problems, consider the following interventions:

- Maintain the airway using manual, basic, and advanced airway devices if needed.
- Position the patient appropriately to decrease the risk of aspiration.
- Do not give the patient anything to eat or drink initially.
  - Assess the patient's gag reflex.
- Administer oxygen to maintain $SaO_2 > 92\%$.
- Assist ventilation if needed.
- Be prepared to suction the airway.

Seizures

In some patients, the postictal state after a seizure can mimic the signs or symptoms of stroke. Seizures may also occur as a result of stroke, although they rarely occur after thrombotic strokes. Treat recurrent seizures to prevent further deterioration of your patient.
Treat patients as follows:

- Maintain the airway.
- Administer oxygen.
- Protect the patient from injury.
- Administer anticonvulsant drugs:
  - Diazepam, lorazepam, or midazolam
- Then administer longer-acting anticonvulsants:
  - Phenytoin, fosphenytoin, or phenobarbital

Emergency Management of Hypertension Before tPA in Acute Ischemic Stroke

In acute ischemic stroke, the emergency management of hypertension prior to tPA is controversial. It includes the following:

- Pre-tPA hypertension control
  - Do not treat BP if SBP is < 185 mmHg or DBP < 110 mmHg.

- If SBP > 185 mmHg or DBP > 110 mmHg on repeated measurements, treat with:
  - 10- to 20-mg doses of labetalol IVP (may repeat once)
  OR
  - 1–2 inches of nitropaste

Emergency Management of Hypertension Following tPA in Acute Ischemic Stroke

If the patient becomes hypertensive during or after fibrinolytic therapy for an acute ischemic stroke, consider the following:

- If DBP > 140 mmHg on repeated measurements:
  - Administer nitroprusside, 0.5 mcg/kg/min IV infusion.
  - Titrate the dose to achieve the desired DBP.
  - Monitor BP every 15 minutes during nitroprusside infusion; observe for hypotension.
- If SBP > 230 mmHg or if DBP ranges from 121 mmHg to 140 mmHg on repeated measurements:
  - Administer labetalol, 10 mg IVP over 1–2 minutes.
    - If needed, repeat or double labetalol every 10 minutes up to 150 mg.
  - Alternatively, give the initial labetalol bolus and then start a labetalol IV infusion at 2–8 mg/min.
  - Monitor BP every 15 minutes during labetalol administration; observe for hypotension.
  - If there is an unsatisfactory response, infuse nitroprusside 0.5 mcg/kg/min IV and continue monitoring BP.
- If SBP is 180–230 mmHg or if DBP is 105–120 mmHg for two readings 5–10 minutes apart:
  - Administer labetalol, 10 mg IVP over 1–2 minutes.
    - If needed, repeat or double labetalol every 10–20 minutes up to 150 mg.
  - Alternatively, give the initial labetalol bolus and then start a labetalol IV infusion at 2–8 mg/min.
  - Monitor BP every 15 minutes during labetalol administration; observe for hypotension.

The Bottom Line

Follow inclusion and exclusion criteria for tPA administration closely to correctly identify appropriate candidates for treatment and to minimize harm. Few patients meet the inclusion criteria for fibrinolytic therapy following stroke. The window of opportunity to treat those few patients with fibrinolytics is very small. Every member of the emergency care team must act quickly to recognize stroke, initiate appropriate diagnostic tests, and deliver emergency care to patients who have symptoms of stroke.

2

ACLS for Experienced Providers

8

Advanced Acute Coronary Syndromes

> **Chapter 6 discussed early management of ACS** and specific interventions you will employ when caring for patients with ST-segment-elevation myocardial infarction (STEMI). This chapter will describe:
>
> - How to assess and manage patients who present with ACS without STEMI
> - Complications association with myocardial infarction
> - Non-ACS causes of chest pain

Unstable Angina and Non-ST-Segment-Elevation MI (UA/NSTEMI)

Unstable angina (UA) and non-ST-segment-elevation MI (NSTEMI) are part of the continuum of ACS. In patients with these syndromes, there is an increased incidence of death related to heart disease and of myocardial infarction. Patients who have UA/NSTEMI are symptomatic because not enough oxygen is getting to the myocardial tissues to supply the tissue demands.

Unstable Angina (UA)

Unstable angina is most often caused by atherosclerotic coronary artery disease (CAD). The coronary arteries narrow but are not completely occluded. This can occur as a result of a thrombus, an arterial spasm, or an arterial inflammation, or it may be related to an extrinsic cause. Unstable angina does not cause myocardial necrosis; therefore, cardiac biomarkers are not elevated in these patients.

There are three presentations of unstable angina:

1. Angina that occurs at rest lasting > 20 minutes
2. New-onset angina
3. Increasing angina symptoms or frequency

Symptoms of Angina

The characteristics of typical anginal pain are:

- Chest or arm discomfort associated with stress or exertion
  - Pain may be "deep"
  - The patient may have difficulty describing the exact location
- Relief of symptoms with rest and/or nitroglycerin

Anginal Equivalents

Sometimes angina does not present with chest pain. Other symptoms that occur in the same pattern and suggest angina are referred to as "anginal equivalents." These patients may experience discomfort in the ear, jaw, neck, arm, or epigastric area. Occasionally patients with UA will present without any discomfort. These atypical features are more common in women, diabetics, and old patients. Their symptoms may include:

- Exertional dyspnea that is new or unexplained
- Nausea, vomiting
- Diaphoresis

The pace and intensity with which the patient's symptoms have been escalating will influence your decision making. Questions such as "Did this pain awake you from sleep?" can provide very significant information about the tempo of the angina.

Non-ST-Segment-Elevation MI (NSTEMI)

The signs and symptoms of unstable angina and NSTEMI are similar; however, there is an important pathologic difference. Myocardial necrosis occurs in patients with NSTEMI because the hypoxic episode was sufficiently long and severe. Cardiac biomarkers will be elevated in patients with NSTEMI. These patients do not initially have ST-segment elevation on the 12-lead ECG and most are later diagnosed with a non-Q-wave myocardial infarction.

Patients with unstable angina and non-ST-segment-elevation MI follow the same treatment path.

Risk Estimation

Patients should be sorted into risk categories that identify the likelihood that the symptoms are related to CAD and that predict the chance of an adverse outcome. This risk estimation is based on patient age, history, symptoms, physical findings, the ECG interpretation, and the measurement of cardiac markers (Table 8-1). Braunwald et al. have developed several tools to help clinicians identify patients who are more likely to have chest pain caused by coronary artery disease. Assigning a risk category can also help you determine the appropriate location for patient care and the type of treatment needed. Risk categories should be used within the context of the other elements of the physical exam and the clinical course.

TABLE 8-1 Likelihood That Signs and Symptoms Represent an ACS Secondary to CAD

	A. High Likelihood	**B. Intermediate Likelihood**	**C. Low Likelihood**
History	Chest or left-arm pain or discomfort as chief symptom, reproducing prior documented angina Known history of CAD, including MI	Chest or left-arm pain or discomfort as chief symptom Age > 70 years Male sex Diabetes mellitus	Probable ischemic symptoms in absence of any of the intermediate likelihood characteristics Recent cocaine use
Examination	Transient MR, hypotension, diaphoresis, pulmonary edema or rales	Extracardiac vascular disease	Chest discomfort reproduced by palpation
ECG	New (or presumably new) transient ST-segment deviation (≥ 0.05 mV) or T-wave inversion (≥ 0.2 mV) with symptoms	Fixed Q waves Abnormal ST segments or T waves not documented to be new	T-wave flattening or inversion in leads with dominant R waves Normal ECG
Cardiac markers	Elevated TnI, TnT, or CK-MB	Normal	Normal

Source: Borrowed with permission from E. Braunwald et al., "ACC/AHA 2002 Guideline Update for the Management of Patients with Unstable Angina and Non-ST-Segment Elevation Myocardial Infarction: Summary Article—A Report of the American College of Cardiology/American Heart Association Task Force on Practice Guidelines (Committee on the Management of Patients with Unstable Angina)," *J. Am. Coll. Cardiol.* 40, no. 7 (Oct. 2002): 1366–1374. PMID: 12383588; http://acc.org/clinical/guidelines/unstable/unstable.pdf (accessed 3/20/06).

Risk Calculator for Unstable Angina/ Non-ST-Segment-Elevation MI

The thrombolysis in myocardial infarction (TIMI) risk calculator is a decision tool that will help predict the likelihood of adverse outcomes in patients with unstable angina or non-ST-segment-elevation MI. Patients are categorized as having a low, moderate, or high risk of death; having a new or recurrent MI; or needing urgent revascularization.

Table 8-2 provides information to calculate the risk for unstable angina/non-ST-segment-elevation MI.

TABLE 8-2   Thrombolysis in Myocardial Infarction (TIMI) Risk Score for Unstable Angina/Non-ST-Segment-Elevation MI

Patient History	Points
Age ≥ 65	1
≥ 3 coronary artery disease (CAD) risk factors:	1
■ Family history of CAD	
■ Hypertension	
■ Elevated cholesterol	
■ Diabetes mellitus	
■ Current smoker	
Known CAD (stenosis ≥ 50%)	1
Aspirin use in last 7 days	1
Patient Presentation	
Recent severe angina (≥ 24 hours)	1
■ More than 2 anginal events in 24 hours	
Elevated serum cardiac markers	1
ST-segment deviation ≥ 0.5 mm	1
■ *Or* transient ST-segment elevation < 20 minutes	
Risk Score = Total Points (0–7):	
Risk score 0–2 = low risk	
Risk score 3–4 = intermediate risk	
Risk score 5–7 = high risk	

Source: Adapted with permission from E. M. Antman et al., "The TIMI Risk Score for Unstable Angina/Non-ST-Evaluation MI: A Method for Prognostication and Therapeutic Decision Making," *JAMA* 284, pp. 835-842, 2000.

American College of Cardiologists (ACC)/American Heart Association (AHA) High-Risk Indicators

The ACC and AHA have identified other risk factors to evaluate. If any of these factors is present, place the patient in the high-risk category: [1]

■ Percutaneous coronary intervention (PCI) within 6 months
■ Prior coronary artery bypass graft (CABG)

---

[1]Adapted with permission from E. Braunwald et al., "ACC/AHA 2002 Guidelines Update for the Management of Patients with Unstable Angina and Non-ST-Segment Elevation Myocardial Infarction: Summary Article—A Report of the American College of Cardiology/American Heart Association Task Force on Practice Guidelines (Committee on the Management of Patients with Unstable Angina)," *J. Am. Coll. Cardiol.* 40, no. 7 (Oct. 2002): 1366–1374. PMID: 12383588; available at http://acc.org/clinical/guidelines/unstable/unstable.pdf (accessed 3/20/06).

- Recurrent angina/ischemia with CHF symptoms
  - S-3 gallop
  - Pulmonary edema
  - Increasing rales
  - New or worsening mitral valve regurgitation
- High-risk findings on noninvasive stress testing
- Depressed LV systolic function
  - Ejection fraction < 0.40 on a noninvasive study
- Hemodynamic instability
- Recurrent, nonsustained, or sustained ventricular tachycardia

Care of the Patient with UA/NSTEMI

The appropriate treatment path for patients with UA/STEMI is complex and based upon continual analysis of the patient's symptoms, physical exam, ECG, cardiac markers, and an analysis of risk. This evaluation will lead to a determination that the patient has a high, intermediate, or low risk of UA/NSTEMI. The initial care of all of these patients should include standard emergency care measures.

Algorithm for UA/NSTEMI Risk Stratification

Primary ABCD Survey

↓

O_2; IV; cardiac monitor; assess vital signs; attach pulse oximeter; obtain history, physical exam, 12- or 15-lead ECG promptly, serum cardiac markers, electrolyte and coagulation studies, and portable chest X-ray

↓

Immediate general treatment ("MONA")

- Oxygen 4 L/min
- Aspirin 162–325 mg
- Nitroglycerin SL for ischemic chest pain
- Morphine sulfate IV if pain not relieved with NTG

↓

12-lead ECG interpretation shows ST-segment depression, T-wave inversion, normal ECG, or nondiagnostic ECG

↓

Assess TIMI risk score

↓

Assess for any ACC/AHA high-risk indicators:

↓

Determine Risk:

↓

High Risk
ST deviation
TIMI risk score ≥ 5
Elevated cardiac markers
Unstable angina
ACC/AHA high-risk indictor present

↓

Intermediate Risk
TIMI risk score of 3–4
Age ≥ 75

↓

Low Risk
No high- or intermediate-risk factors identified

◇ ◇ ◇ **Testing Tips**

- Just because the patient has a normal initial 12-lead ECG does not mean that she or he doesn't have a life-threatening ACS. Be sure to look at the whole picture and use the decision-making tools to help determine the patient's risk.

Medical Management of Patients with UA/NSTEMI

Standard measures for ACS (oxygen, aspirin, nitroglycerin, morphine) are given to all patients of ACS during the initial evaluation and are continued if needed during care. Additional medical interventions may be considered during care of all UA/STEMI and are based on the individual patient's needs. General medical management that may be indicated includes the following:

- Nitroglycerin IV
  - If symptoms persist after 3 doses of sublingual NTG and beta-blocker
  - Not indicated if the patient is hypotensive or has recently used erectile dysfunction drugs

- Beta-blocker therapy
  - Slows the heart rate; decreases contractility and systolic BP
    - Reduces myocardial oxygen demand
  - Should be started early
    - Give IV then orally
  - Not indicated in the presence of the following:
    - Heart block, asthma, severe LV dysfunction
    - HR < 50 bpm
    - SBP < 90 mmHg
- Calcium channel blocker treatment
  - Second- or third-line choice for symptom control after nitrates
  - Alternative drug for rate control if beta-blockers cannot be used
  - Use is controversial
- ACE inhibitor administration
  - Helpful in myocardial infarction with:
    - LV dysfunction
    - Diabetic patients with LV dysfunction
    - Other high-risk patients with normal LV function
- Oral administration of HMG coenzyme A reductase inhibitors (statin drugs)
  - Helpful when started within 24 hours of symptom onset

Other interventions will depend on the patient's individual clinical presentation and on the patient's risk stratification.

Algorithm for UA/NSTEMI for High-Risk Patients

The following algorithm presents the initial emergency care and risk stratification for high-risk patients with UA/NSTEMI. For the medical management noted at the beginning of the algorithm, refer to the previous section, "Medical Management of Patients with UA/NSTEMI."

Medical Management
Anticoagulate with UFH or enoxaparin

↓

Early invasive strategy available?

↓

Yes   No

↓   ↓

Positive troponin?   *Early conservative strategy:*
                                                            Add clopidogrel
↓   Admit

GP IIb/IIIa inhibitor infusion   ↓
(eptifibatide or tirofiban)

↓

Early invasive strategy:
Cardiac catheterization

↓

Perform PCI or refer for CABG

↓

Add clopidogrel if PCI and a stent is used

Send to the cath lab if one of more of the following develops:

- Persistent ischemic chest pain
- Recurrent/persistent ST deviation
- Ventricular tachycardia
- Hemodynamic instability
- Signs of pump failure: S-3 gallop, pulmonary edema, increasing rales, new or worsening mitral regurgitation

Algorithm for UA/NSTEMI for Intermediate- or Low-Risk Patients

The following algorithm presents the initial emergency care and risk stratification for intermediate- or low-risk patients with UA/NSTEMI. To review the medical management noted at the beginning of the algorithm, refer to the earlier section, "Medical Management of Patients with UA/NSTEMI."

Risk Level

Intermediate Risk
Medical management

↓

Administer enoxaparin

Low Risk
Medical management

↓

Individualized treatment

↓

Continue the evaluation
Repeat the 12-lead ECG at least twice
Repeat cardiac markers twice ≥ 6–8 hours after the onset of chest pain
Consider immediate cardiac stress test

↓

Do high-risk indicators develop during evaluation?

Yes

↓

Go to early invasive strategy
in high-risk algorithm

No

↓

Discharge

(continued)

TIMI risk score
of 3–4:

- Aspirin
- Consider
  Clopidogrel
- Appointment
  with cardiologist

TIMI risk score
of 0–2:

- Consider
  aspirin
- Appointment
  with primary
  care MD

Complications of Acute Coronary Syndromes

Most patients who develop shock after myocardial infarction have damage to a large area of the left ventricle. The mortality rate in these patients is very high. If the patient presents with shock or pulmonary edema and ST-segment-elevation MI, PCI is the preferred reperfusion therapy. If you are in a facility without PCI, a fibrinolytic drug should be given if the delay for PCI will be longer than 60 minutes. The patient should then be transferred to a hospital where the procedure can be performed. Fibrinolytic treatment is not indicated if the patient has UA/NSTEMI. Treat the patient's signs and symptoms until definitive care can be given. If the patient presents with shock, deliver care using the Algorithm for Hypotension/Shock. To manage acute pulmonary edema, follow the Algorithm for Acute Pulmonary Edema.

Algorithm for Hypotension/Shock

▶ Primary ABCD survey

▶ O₂; IV; cardiac monitor; assess vital signs; attach pulse oximeter; obtain history, physical exam, 12-lead ECG, and portable chest X-ray

▶ Rate problem?
▶ Bradycardia—see Bradycardia Algorithm (Chapter 5)
▶ Tachycardia—see appropriate Tachycardia Algorithm (Chapter 5)

▶ Volume problem?
- Give IV fluids, blood transfusion (if appropriate)
- Consider vasopressors
- Treat specific cause if identified

▶ Pump problem?
- Consider fluid bolus of 250–500 mL normal saline (if lungs are clear)
- SBP < 70 mmHg
  - Norepinephrine IV infusion 0.5–30 mcg/min
- SBP 70–100 mmHg
  - With signs and symptoms of shock—dopamine, IV infusion 2–20 mcg/kg/min
  - Without signs and symptoms of shock—dobutamine, IV infusion 2–20 mcg/kg/min

▶ Consider:
- Pulmonary artery catheter
- Intra-aortic balloon pump
- Angiography for acute MI/ischemia
- Additional diagnostic studies
- Surgical repair (select conditions)

Source: Antman, E. M., Anbe, D. T., Armstrong, P. W., Bates, E. R., Green, L. A., Hand, M., Hochman, J. S., Krumholz, H. M., Kushner, F. G., Lamas, G. A., Mullany, C. J., Ornato, J. P., Pearle, D. L., Sloan, M. A., Smith, S. C., Jr., ACC/AHA guidelines for the management of patients with ST-elevation myocardial infarction: executive summary: a report of the ACC/AHA Task Force on Practice Guidelines (Committee to Revise the 1999 Guidelines on the Management of Patients with Acute Myocardial Infarction.) *Circulation.* 2004; 110:588–636.

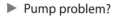

◆ ◆ ◆ Testing Tips

■ When the patient's blood pressure is low, don't automatically react by giving a fluid bolus. First, evaluate the situation based on the patient's history and physical exam. Then decide if the hypotension is caused by a rate problem, a volume problem, or a pump problem. After you make that determination, you can choose the appropriate intervention.

Algorithm for Acute Pulmonary Edema

▶ Primary ABCD survey

▶ O_2; IV; cardiac monitor; assess vital signs; attach pulse oximeter; obtain history, physical exam, 12-lead ECG, and portable chest X-ray

(continued)

▶ Initial actions:
- Oxygen, intubation if needed; initiate continuous positive airway pressure (CPAP) or bi-level positive airway pressure (BiPAP)
- Nitroglycerin, 0.4 mg SL
- Furosemide, 0.5–1.0 mg/kg IVP
- Morphine sulfate, 2–4 mg IV

↓

▶ Secondary actions:
- Nitroglycerin or nitroprusside: IV infusion (start at 10–20 mcg/min and increase dose 5 mcg/min every 5–10 minutes to desired effect) if SBP > 100 mmHg
- Dopamine: 2–20 mcg/kg/min IV infusion if SBP 70–100 mmHg with shock signs and symptoms
- Dobutamine: 2–20 mcg/kg/min IV infusion if SBP > 100 mmHg with no shock signs and symptoms

↓

▶ Consider:
- Pulmonary artery catheter
- Intra-aortic balloon pump
- Angiography for acute MI/ischemia
- Additional diagnostic studies
- Consider treatment with ACE inhibitors

Atypical Acute Coronary Syndromes

Some patients who are having an acute coronary syndrome experience atypical symptoms (Table 8-3). Failure to consider this during initial triage, transport, or care of your patient can be a critical error.

Causes of Chest Pain That Mimic ACS

A significant number of conditions that are not ACS will initially present with symptoms of ACS. Perform a careful history, physical exam, and diagnostic testing to distinguish between these conditions so that you can provide appropriate patient care. Table 8-4 categorizes causes of chest pain that mimic ACS.

Causes and Differential Diagnoses of Chest Pain

Some noncardiac diseases present with chest pain. Table 8-5 outlines characteristic features of diseases that present with chest pain and suggests diagnostic tests that will help you distinguish between them.

TABLE 8-3   Atypical Acute Coronary Syndromes

Patient Population	Atypical Signs and Symptoms
Diabetics	■ Instead of typical angina, the diabetic patient may have shortness of breath, diaphoresis, gastrointestinal complaints, weakness, syncope, or profound fatigue. ■ The diabetic patient may experience discomfort in unusual locations and with abnormal descriptions.
Elderly	■ The elderly patient may present with acute weakness, syncope, confusion, unexplained sinus tachycardia, bronchospasm due to cardiogenic asthma, new-onset lower extremity edema, shortness of breath, fatigue, and/or abdominal or epigastric discomfort.
Women	■ In addition to the chest pain and difficulty breathing that both women and men experience, women are more likely than men are to present with mid-back pain, nausea and/or vomiting, palpitations, and indigestion.[2]

[2]K. A. Milner, M. Funk, S. Richards, R. Wilmes, V. Vaccarino, and H. M. Krumholz, "Gender Differences in Symptom Presentation Associated with Coronary Heart Disease," *Am. J. Cardiol.* 84, no. 4 (Aug. 1999): 396–399. PMID: 10468075.

TABLE 8-4   Non-ACS Causes of Chest Pain

Degree of Severity	Non-ACS Conditions
Life-threatening	■ Aortic dissection ■ Pericardial effusion and tamponade ■ Pulmonary embolism ■ Pneumothorax
Serious, with potential for significant morbidity	■ Perforated peptic ulcer, cholecystitis, pancreatitis ■ Esophageal rupture ■ Pneumonia ■ Aortic stenosis
Less potential for immediate morbidity	■ Gastroesophageal reflux disease (GERD) ■ Esophagitis, gastritis ■ Hiatal hernia ■ Musculoskeletal causes, including costochondritis

TABLE 8-5 Causes and Differential Diagnoses of Chest Pain

Diagnosis	Signs/Symptoms	Useful Tests
Acute coronary syndrome	■ Retrosternal pressure that may radiate to the neck, jaw, both arms, upper back, epigastrium, and sides of chest (left more than right) ■ Chest pain with dyspnea, nausea, vomiting, diaphoresis	■ 12-lead ECG ■ Serum markers (troponins, CK-MB)
Aortic dissection (thoracic)	■ Abrupt onset of severe pain described as tearing, ripping, or knifelike in the anterior chest, often radiating to the back between the shoulder blades ■ May have unequal pulses and blood pressures in the upper extremities	■ CXR ■ CT scan ■ Transthoracic ultrasound ■ Transesophageal ultrasound ■ MRI ■ 12-lead ECG
Pericarditis	■ Dull, aching, recurrent pain unrelated to exercise or meals, or sharp, stabbing retrosternal pain that may radiate to the left shoulder ■ May last hours to days and may be episodic ■ Pain is often worse when supine, better when sitting up ■ Friction rub may be heard	■ 12-lead ECG ■ Echocardiogram ■ CT scan ■ MRI
Pulmonary embolism	■ Sudden onset (pleuritic in nature), dyspnea, tachypnea, tachycardia, hypotension, anxiety, possible pleural rub, syncope, hemoptysis	■ Angiography ■ CXR ■ ECG ■ Spiral CT scan ■ ABG ■ Ventilation-perfusion scan
Pneumothorax	■ Sudden-onset severe pain (pleuritic in nature), dyspnea, decreased breath sounds, decreased chest expansion, hypoxemia ■ Hypotension, possible jugular venous distension, and altered mental status with tension pneumothorax	■ CXR ■ CT scan
Peptic ulcer	■ Epigastric, substernal pain relieved with food or antacids	■ Endoscopy

Acute cholecystitis	■ Burning ■ Pressure located in the right upper quadrant or epigastrium ■ May radiate to right scapula ■ May follow meal	■ Abdominal ultrasound ■ CT scan ■ Liver function tests
Pancreatitis	■ Steady mid-epigastric pain with radiation to back ■ Nausea, vomiting, tachycardia	■ Amylase/lipase ■ Abdominal ultrasound ■ CT scan
Esophageal rupture	■ Abrupt onset of retrosternal pain, usually preceded by vomiting ■ Pain radiates to the back or epigastrium and is increased by swallowing or neck flexion ■ Melena, hematemesis, tachycardia	■ CXR ■ Water-soluble contrast esophagram or esophagoscopy
Pneumonia	■ Unilateral, often localized pain ■ Dyspnea, cough, fever	■ CXR ■ CBC
Aortic stenosis	■ Chest pain, syncope, exertional dyspnea	■ Echocardiogram ■ Cardiac catheterization
Gastroesophageal reflux disease	■ Chest pain, retrosternal burning sensation most commonly occurring after a meal ■ Difficult and/or painful swallowing	■ Endoscopy ■ Upper GI
Esophagitis, gastritis	■ Chest pain described as a "burning" sensation ■ Abdominal pain, nausea, vomiting ■ Esophageal pain that is often positional and related to swallowing	■ Upper GI series ■ Esophageal manometry, esophagoscopy, or gastroscopy
Hiatal hernia	■ Dull discomfort, localized pressure, or severe squeezing pain across the middle of the chest	■ Upper GI series ■ Esophageal manometry or esophagoscopy
Musculoskeletal cause, including costochondritis, muscle strain, intercostal strain, rib fracture	■ Usually tender over a specific point that reproduces pain ■ Aggravated by movement	■ Diagnosis of exclusion once risk factors have been assessed

The Bottom Line

Many patients with chest pain do not have a "classic" clinical picture of acute myocardial infarction that includes obvious ST-segment elevation on the 12-lead ECG. Deciding on the appropriate plan of care can be a challenge in these cases. Using evidence-based strategies to differentiate low-risk from high-risk patients with ACS and to distinguish non-cardiac causes of chest pain will help you provide the safest, most reliable care to these patients.

9

Toxicology in ACLS

In 2002, there were more than 2 million cases of human exposures to poison reported to the American Association of Poison Control Centers.[1] Drugs involved in the most frequent causes of death from ingested poisons are antidepressants, and street drugs (including cocaine and heroin), opiates, and cardiovascular drugs. For each person who dies from toxic poisoning, there are about 150 who have nonfatal poison exposures. Of those 150, some have no symptoms while others have life-threatening signs or symptoms and are hospitalized in intensive care units.

Toxicology Resources

When you encounter a patient who has been poisoned, consult a medical toxicologist or certified regional poison information center. Expert advice is desirable when you treat poisoned patients with life-threatening signs or symptoms related to their toxic exposure. They may need a specialized antidote or higher doses of medications than usual to manage their signs or symptoms. In the United States, the national Poison Control number is 1-800-222-1222.

If a medical toxicologist or certified regional poison information center is not available to you, consult printed reference materials to ensure that you follow the proper treatment plan.

Airway Management

Poisoned patients can deteriorate rapidly, so frequent reassessment of their airway and breathing is essential. It is important to obtain arterial blood gasses to assess oxygenation, ventilation, and the presence of acidosis in some poisoned patients.

If the patient's airway and ventilation are severely impaired due to an overdose of opiates, ventilate the patient immediately. Then administer an opioid antagonist (naloxone or nalmefene) *before* intubating the patient. If the patient responds to the narcotic antagonist, intubation will rarely be needed. When using naloxone or nalmefene, the

---

[1] American Association of Poison Control Centers, www.aapcc.org/2002_poison_surve_results.htm.

recommended endpoint is arousal of the patient to the point where adequate airway reflexes and ventilation are present, but not complete alertness. Acute withdrawal may be avoided by titrating the dose of antagonist and leaving the patient somewhat sedated. The effects of narcotics often outlast the antagonistic effects of naloxone by 2 or more hours. Monitor the patient closely after administration to assess the need for additional doses of naloxone.

Benzodiazepine antagonists may be given to reverse airway depression after procedural sedation. They are not recommended for routine use in patient overdose. Serious side effects can occur if the patient is dependent on benzodiazepines, has a seizure disorder, or has taken tricyclic antidepressant drugs.

Rapid sequence intubation (RSI) is recommended before performing gastric lavage in an obtunded or comatose patient.

Prolonged CPR

Prolonged CPR (> 1 hour) may be warranted in some poisoned patients, particularly in those who have had a witnessed cardiac arrest or in those with calcium channel blocker overdose.

Tachycardias

Tachycardias that result from poisoning can lead to:

- Myocardial ischemia
- Myocardial infarction
- Ventricular arrhythmias
- Heart failure
- Shock

Benzodiazepines such as diazepam or lorazepam may be useful in the management of sympathomimetic-induced chest pain, hypertension, or tachycardia. Avoid using benzodiazepines in amounts that result in deep sedation or the need for respiratory assistance.

Physostigmine (Antilirium) is indicated for hemodynamically significant tachycardia associated with pure anticholinergic poisoning. Do not administer physostigmine if the patient has taken a tricyclic antidepressant overdose. The side effects of physostigmine use include:

- Copious secretions of the lower airways
- Seizures
- Bradycardia
- Asystole

Avoid calcium channel blockers such as verapamil and diltiazem in poisoned patients with borderline hypotension. Using these drugs may result in severe hypotension.

Ventricular Tachycardia/Ventricular Fibrillation

When you treat a patient with stimulant toxicity who is in pulseless ventricular tachycardia or ventricular fibrillation, administer epinephrine in standard doses and increase the interval between doses.

Bradycardias

Bradycardia related to poisoning may not respond to standard emergency cardiac care. In some cases, larger doses of standard drugs are needed. In other cases, a specific antidote will need to be given.

- Severe poisoning by digoxin, calcium channel blockers, or beta-blockers causes severe bradycardia. Atropine may be ineffective to treat these patients, even in high doses.
- If hemodynamically significant bradycardia does not respond to atropine and pacing, consider administering high-dose vasopressor therapy or the use of a circulatory assist device.
- Atropine is indicated in higher than normal doses to treat poisoning from organophosphates, carbamates, and nerve agents.
- Isoproterenol may be helpful to treat bradycardia resulting from beta-blocker overdose. Do not give isoproterenol if the bradycardia is caused by anticholinesterase poisoning. In general, isoproterenol should be used rarely in patients with toxic poisoning.

Systemic Alkalinization

When systemic alkalinization is necessary in specific severe poisonings, try to achieve an arterial pH of 7.50–7.55. If the patient has overdosed on a sodium channel antagonist, alkalinization will prevent or reverse supraventricular tachycardias with aberrant conduction and ventricular tachycardia. Consider administration of sodium bicarbonate for alkalinization if the patient has had a toxic exposure of tricyclic antidepressants or cocaine.

Gastric Decontamination

Activated charcoal is the preferred method of GI decontamination if the patient presents within 1 hour of the ingestion. Multiple-dose charcoal may be beneficial. Other methods include the following:

- Gastric lavage is indicated only if the ingestion is known to have occurred less than 1 hour prior.
- Whole bowel irrigation may be considered. It involves flushing the GI tract with a nonabsorbable isotonic electrolyte solution containing polyethylene glycol. Have the patient drink the solution or administer it through a nasogastric tube. Whole bowel irrigation may be useful after the ingestion of enteric-coated or time-released medications (e.g., verapamil).[2]
- Syrup of ipecac should not be used to treat poisoned patients.

Shock

Drug-induced shock is usually related to a decrease in intravascular volume, systemic vascular resistance (SVR), myocardial contractility, or a combination of these factors.

---

[2] J.R. Brubacher, "B-Adrenergic Antagonists," in *Goldfrank's Toxicologic Emergencies,* 7th ed., ed. J.R. Goldfrank (McGraw-Hill, 2002).

Drug-Induced Hypovolemic Shock

If you suspect drug-induced hypovolemic shock in a patient with normal systemic vascular resistance, administer a fluid challenge. Patients poisoned with cardiotoxic agents may not tolerate a large-volume IV fluid infusion. It can lead to fluid overload and congestive heart failure. If shock persists despite adequate fluid administration, administer a vasopressor.

Drug-Induced Distributive Shock

Patients with drug-induced distributive shock have a normal or high cardiac output, but very low systemic vascular resistance. To put it simply, the heart is pumping fast enough and forcefully enough and there is plenty of fluid in the body—the containers (blood vessels) are just larger. You may need to administer high-dose vasopressor therapy when drug-induced distributive shock does not respond to standard vasopressor therapy.

Drug-Induced Cardiogenic Shock

Administer inotropic agents in cases of drug-induced shock characterized by a low cardiac output and high SVR. Inotropic agents to consider in severely poisoned patients include inamrinone, dobutamine, calcium, glucagon, and norepinephrine.

 # Toxidromes

A toxidrome is a group of signs and symptoms that indicate a specific class of poisoning (Table 9-1). Understanding signs and symptoms of each toxidrome and the specific interventions used to treat them can be helpful when the exact source of poisoning is unknown. Toxidromes include anticholinergic, cholinergic, opiate, sedative/hypnotic, and sympathomimetic.

TABLE 9-1 Common Toxidromes

Toxidrome Causative Agents	Signs and Symptoms	Interventions to Consider
Anticholinergic Antihistamines, antipsychotics, antidepressants, antispasmodics, atropine, jimson weed, phenothiazines, scopolamine	Delirium, memory loss, flushing, tachycardia, supraventricular arrhythmias, ventricular arrhythmias, impaired conduction, shock, cardiac arrest, urinary retention, dry skin, elevated temperature, hypertension, blurred vision, dilated pupils, decreased bowel sounds, psychosis, hallucinations, seizures, coma	■ Maintain the airway ■ Monitor the patient ■ Administer physostigmine

Cholinergic Carbamates, some mushrooms, nerve agents, organophosphates, physostigmine	Excessive secretions, vomiting, and diarrhea; bradycardia or ventricular arrhythmias; impaired conduction; shock; bronchorrhea; bronchospasm; miosis; muscle fasciculations; pulmonary edema; seizures	▪ Decontaminate the patient if indicated ▪ Protect the airway/provide suction ▪ Manage the airway ▪ Administer high-dose atropine ▪ Administer pralidoxime ▪ Treat seizures with benzodiazepines
Opiate Dextromethorphan, heroin, morphine, fentanyl, oxycodone, oxycontin, propoxyphene, others	Altered mental status, pinpoint pupils, bradycardia, unresponsiveness, shallow respirations, slow respiratory rate, decreased bowel sounds, hypothermia, hypotension, respiratory arrest	▪ Open the airway ▪ Assist with ventilation ▪ Administer naloxone dose to restore airway reflexes ▪ Consider intubation ▪ Consider nalmefene
Sedative/hypnotic Anticonvulsants, barbiturates, benzodiazepines, ethanol	Confusion, respiratory depression, hypotension, decreased temperature, confusion, delirium, hallucinations, coma, paresthesias, blurred vision, slurred speech, ataxia, nystagmus	▪ Maintain the airway ▪ Ventilate if necessary ▪ Administer IV fluids if hypotensive ▪ Administer flumazenil if the toxicity results from benzodiazepine use during procedural sedation

Sympathomimetic
Amphetamines, cocaine, ephedrine, methamphetamine, phencyclidine, pseudoephedrine
	Restlessness, anxiety or delirium, excessive speech and motor activity, tremor, dilated pupils, disorientation, insomnia, tachycardia, hallucinations, hypertensive crisis, ventricular dysrhythmias, acute coronary syndromes, shock, cardiac arrest, possible seizures or stroke, hyperthermia	▪ Maintain the airway
		▪ Administer:
		  ▪ Benzodiazepines (for arrhythmias seizures or chest pain)
		  ▪ Sodium bicarbonate (used to treat ventricular arrhythmias if cocaine used)
		  ▪ Lidocaine
		  ▪ Nitroglycerin (for ACS)
		▪ In ACS, angioplasty is preferred over fibrinolytics
		▪ Avoid beta-blockers
		▪ Do *NOT* use propranolol if cocaine toxicity
		▪ Cooling measures

◇ ◇ ◇ **Testing Tips**

There are a couple of mnemonics that can help you recognize the signs and symptoms of some toxidromes:

- For anticholinergic toxicity, think of "Hot as Hades, red as a beet, dry as a bone, blind as a bat, mad as a hatter":

    "Hot as Hades" (increased temperature)

    "Red as a beet" (flushed skin)

    "Dry as a bone" (decreased salivation)

    "Blind as a bat" (dilated pupils)

    "Mad as a hatter" (delirium)

- For cholinergic poisonings, remember "SLUDGE"

    Salivation

    Lacrimation

    Urination

    Defecation

    GI distress (cramping)

    Emesis

Beta-Blocker Toxicity

The effects of beta-blocker overdose usually begin within ½ hour following an overdose and peak within 2 hours. Onset may be delayed with the ingestion of sustained-release preparations.[3]

The signs and symptoms of toxic beta-blocker overdose include:

- Altered mental status
- Bradycardia
    - Prolonged QRS and QT interval
- Hypotension
- Hypoglycemia (more common in children)

Treatment of Beta-Blocker Toxicity

Begin treatment of the patient with a beta-blocker overdose with an initial assessment and ECG monitoring. Specific interventions for these patients include:

- High-dose vasopressors
    - Epinephrine 2–10 mcg/min. infusion

---

[3] J. R. Brubacher, "B-Adrenergic Antagonists," in *Goldfrank's Toxicologic Emergencies,* 7th ed., ed. J. R. Goldfrank (McGraw-Hill, 2002).

- Gastric decontamination with activated charcoal if the patient presents within 1 hour of the ingestion
- Infusion of 500–1000 mL of isotonic IV fluid if the patient is hypotensive[4]
  - Monitor closely for development of pulmonary edema
- Assessment of blood glucose
  - Treat hypoglycemia
- Glucagon
  - Has inotropic and chronotropic effects and helps counteract hypoglycemia induced by beta-blocker overdose
- Atropine
  - May be used to treat hemodynamically significant bradycardia, but may quickly wear off or become ineffective
- Transcutaneous pacing
- Calcium salts
  - Weak evidence supports the use of calcium
- Extracorporeal membrane oxygenation (ECMO)
  - May be beneficial if the ingested beta-blocker was water soluble and if all other measures are unsuccessful

Calcium Channel Blocker Toxicity

Toxic effects related to a calcium channel blocker overdose begin within 2 hours of the ingestion of immediate-release preparations, but may be delayed up to 5 hours following overdoses of sustained-release preparations.[5] Patients may present with the following signs and symptoms:

- Bradycardia
  - SA and AV node effects
- Impaired conduction
- Shock
  - Hypotension
  - Vasodilation
  - Impaired myocardial contractility
- Altered mental status
  - Related to poor cerebral perfusion
  - Syncope, seizures, coma
- Pulmonary edema
- Hyperglycemia
- Illeus

---

[4] Ibid.

[5] F. De Roos, "Calcium Channel Blockers," in *Goldfrank's Toxicologic Emergencies,* 7th ed., ed. J. R. Goldfrank (McGraw-Hill, 2002).

Treatment of Calcium Channel Blocker Toxicity

Begin treatment of calcium channel blocker toxicity with the assessment and management of the patient's airway, breathing, and circulation. Toxicity-specific interventions include:

- Infusion of 500–1000 mL of isotonic IV fluid for hypotension
  - Monitor the patient closely for pulmonary edema
- Monitor the ECG
  - Frequently evaluate the atrial rate, the ventricular rate, and the PR, QRS, and QT intervals
  - Perform serial 12-lead ECGs
- Gastric emptying or activated charcoal
  - May be beneficial within 1 hour of ingestion
- Whole bowel irrigation
  - Consider for ingestion of sustained-release preparations if severe toxicity is anticipated[6]
- Other possible interventions:
  - May treat hemodynamically significant bradycardia with:
    - Atropine or glucagon
    - Calcium chloride
    - Pacing (external or internal)
- High-dose vasopressors
- High-dose insulin
  - Can be given with glucose and potassium to improve myocardial metabolism and contractility
- Intra-aortic balloon pump support
  - Consider for patients with refractory shock.

Cardiac Glycoside Toxicity

Digitalis preparation toxicity is a common drug-related poisoning. Overdose often results from unintentional toxicity or medication errors. The toxic effects of cardiac glycosides are numerous and include the following:

- Cardiac rhythm disturbances
  - Ventricular arrhythmias
  - AV blocks
  - Sinus bradycardia
  - Atrial arrhythmias
  - Cardiac arrest

---

[6] Ibid.

- Gastrointestinal upset
  - Nausea, vomiting, diarrhea
  - Abdominal pain
- Neurologic symptoms
  - Dizziness, fatigue
  - Confusion, disorientation
  - Altered thought processes
  - Visual alterations
  - Aphasia
  - Seizures

Possible Interventions

The treatment of cardiac glycoside toxicity is based on two principles. First, try to retard absorption or promote elimination of the drug from the body. Second, treat the symptoms and try to prevent life-threatening effects of the toxicity. When caring for a patient who has a digitalis overdose, you may:

- Administer activated charcoal if the patient presents within 1 hour of the ingestion.
- Pretreat with atropine before procedures such as tracheal or gastric intubation to avoid increased vagal tone.
- Correct hypoxia and electrolyte abnormalities (e.g., potassium, magnesium, and calcium).
- Administer normal saline to correct any fluid volume deficit.
- Treat hemodynamically significant bradycardia with atropine and possibly phenytoin.
- Attempt pacing with caution—it may cause ventricular arrhythmias.

Management of Ventricular Tachyarrhythmias

- Digitalis-induced unstable VT:
  - Synchronized cardioversion. Start with low energy levels of 25–50 J. If no response, shock with 200 J (or appropriate biphasic energy). If no response, shock with 300 J (or appropriate biphasic energy).
  - Administer 10–20 vials of digoxin immune fab antibodies. (Each vial can neutralize 0.6 mg of digoxin.)
    - The onset of action is within 1 hour.
  - Give lidocaine 1.5 mg/kg IVP.
    - If the rhythm converts, administer a continuous lidocaine infusion of 1–4 mg/min until Fab-fragment therapy becomes effective.
  - If VT continues after the lidocaine bolus, give magnesium sulfate 1–2 g IVP diluted in 10 mL D5W over 1–2 minutes.

- If the patient's rhythm converts to sinus rhythm after administration of lidocaine and magnesium, infuse magnesium 1–2 g diluted in 50–100 mL D5W over 30–60 minutes.
- Digitalis-induced VF/pulseless VT:
  - Defibrillate 120–200 biphasic; 360 J monophasic.
  - Continue CPR, intubate, and start an IV.
  - Administer epinephrine 1 mg IVP every 3–5 minutes.
    - May substitute vasopressin 40 units IVP to replace first or second epinephrine dose
  - Defibrillate with the same or higher energy level.
  - Give lidocaine 1.0–1.5 mg/kg IVP.
  - Give magnesium sulfate 1–2 g IV/IO diluted in 10 mL D5W.
  - Give digoxin immune fab antibodies (an average dose is 10 vials; may need up to 20).
  - If ventricular fibrillation continues, give:
    - Magnesium sulfate, 1–2 g IV/IO diluted in 10 mL D5W; repeat every minute to a maximum dose of 5–10 g.
    - Lidocaine, 0.5–0.75 mg/kg IV/IO; repeat every 8–10 minutes up to 3 mg/kg.[7]

Cocaine Toxicity

The toxic dose of cocaine varies and depends on the amount and route of administration, the presence of other drugs, and individual tolerance.

A patient who has ingested or injected a toxic dose of cocaine may present with:

- Central nervous signs and symptoms
  - Exhilaration
  - Hallucinations
  - Hyperthermia
  - Seizures
  - Stroke
- Cardiac signs and symptoms
  - Acute coronary syndrome
  - Ventricular arrhythmias
  - Decreased myocardial contractility
- Vascular signs and symptoms
  - Increased systemic vascular resistance
  - Hypertension

---

[7] American Heart Association, *ACLS for Experienced Providers* (2003).

Possible Interventions

General interventions to care for a patient with cocaine toxicity begin with management of airway, breathing, and circulation. Correct an elevated body temperature with passive cooling measures such as cold packs to the axilla and groin. Sponge the patient with cool water and use fans to accelerate evaporation. Antipyretics are ineffective.

Management of Cocaine-Induced ACS

- Administer oxygen, aspirin, and nitroglycerin.
- Give a titrated dose of a benzodiazepine:
  - Diazepam, lorazepam, or midazolam
- Administer morphine to treat persistent pain.
- Magnesium may be used because of its beneficial role in acute MI and antispasmodic effects.
- PCI is possibly better than fibrinolytic therapy for presumed cocaine-associated MI.

Management of Cocaine-Induced Tachyarrhythmias

- Benzodiazepines are first-line agents for supraventricular tachyarrhythmias.
- Use beta-blockers cautiously:
  - They may worsen cocaine-induced vasoconstriction.
  - Do *NOT* use propranolol to treat a patient with cocaine toxicity.
- The use of lidocaine for ventricular arrhythmias refractory to benzodiazepines is controversial.
  - It may increase the risk of seizures.

Management of Cocaine-Induced VF/Pulseless VT

- Routine management for pulseless arrest
- Lidocaine
- Give sodium bicarbonate 1 mEq/kg IVP.
  - Used to treat the acidosis that is common to this condition

Tricyclic Antidepressants

An overdose of tricyclic antidepressants (TCAs) can quickly cause a life-threatening situation. The signs and symptoms of TCA overdose can include:

- Central nervous system
  - Agitation, hallucinations
  - Dizziness, sleepiness
  - Decreased level of consciousness, coma
  - Seizures

- Cardiovascular
  - Prolongation of the QRS complex (> 0.12 seconds), an R wave greater than the S wave or > 3 mm in lead aVR, or terminal (last 40 ms) QRS right-axis deviation in the frontal plane (limb leads)
  - Sinus tachycardia
  - Right bundle branch block
  - VT, VF
  - Prolonged QT interval (can progress to torsades de pointes)
  - Hypotension
- Metabolic/other
  - Acidosis
  - Dry mouth
  - Hyperthermia

Effects generally develop within 30–60 minutes of ingestion and peak within 4–12 hours.

Possible Interventions

- If the level of consciousness is depressed, consider other causes.
  - Give naloxone.
  - Consider administering thiamine.
  - Measure blood glucose and administer dextrose IVP if indicated.
- Consider giving activated charcoal if the patient presents within 1 hour of the ingestion.
- Consider gastric lavage for unresponsive patients (after intubation) and in patients who present within 1 hour of ingestion of a life-threatening quantity of a tricyclic antidepressant.
- Infuse normal saline 500–1000 mL to treat hypotension.
  - If hypotension does not respond to fluid therapy, norepinephrine is recommended.[8]
- Serum alkalinization is indicated for patients who have seizures, hypotension unresponsive to crystalloid infusions, a ventricular arrhythmia, or QRS duration > 0.12 seconds.
  - The goal is to raise the serum pH to between 7.50 and 7.55.
  - Give sodium bicarbonate 1 mEq/kg IVP over 1–2 min.[9]
    - Measure arterial pH often to guide subsequent doses.
      - Sodium bicarbonate administration can induce hypokalemia. Monitor serum potassium closely and provide supplemental potassium as necessary.

[8] L. Teba, F. Schiebel, H. V. Dedhia, and V. A. Lazzell, "Beneficial Effect of Norepinephrine in the Treatment of Circulatory Shock Caused by Tricyclic Antidepressant Overdose," *Am. J. Emerg. Med.* 6, no. 6 (Nov. 1988): 566–568. PMID: 3178947.
[9] F. G. Walter and E. F. Bilden, "Antidepressants," in *Rosen's Emergency Medicine: Concepts and Clinical Practice,* 5th ed., ed.-in-chief J. A. Marx (Mosby, 2002).

- To treat seizures, administer sodium bicarbonate in addition to a benzodiazepine. Alkalinization moves the tricyclic antidepressant into the body's fat stores so that they are released more slowly into the system.
- Sodium bicarbonate administration usually increases the effectiveness of IV benzodiazepines (lorazepam, diazepam) in the treatment of seizures.
- IV midazolam boluses followed by an IV maintenance infusion (1–20 mg/hr) have been used to manage seizures refractory to other benzodiazepines.[10]

[10] A. Kumar and T. P. Bleck, "Intravenous Midazolam for the Treatment of Refractory Status Epilepticus," *Crit. Care. Med.* 20, no. 4 (Apr. 1992): 483–488. PMID: 1559361.

The Bottom Line

To effectively manage life threats associated with drug toxicity, you must adapt your standard approach to these emergencies. If you learn the toxidromes and consult with appropriate experts and references for resources when you care for poisoned patients, you are most likely to effect a favorable outcome.

10

Special Resuscitation Situations

Some illnesses, injuries, and environmental circumstances have life-threatening consequences that, if not properly treated, can lead to cardiac arrest or death. In many of these situations, prompt appropriate interventions can avert their fatal outcome.

 ## Rapid Sequence Intubation (RSI)

Rapid sequence intubation (RSI) is a technique in which a sedative or induction agent is administered and followed immediately with a paralyzing dose of a neuromuscular blocking agent to facilitate rapid tracheal intubation.

The decision to intubate should be based on three criteria:[1]

1. Failure to maintain or protect the airway
2. Failure of ventilation or oxygenation
3. The anticipated need for intubation based on the patient's clinical course and the likelihood of deterioration

RSI Protocol

The general RSI protocol consists of "The Seven Ps":

1. Preparation (zero minus 10 minutes):
   - Assess airway difficulty.
   - Plan the approach.

---

[1] R. M. Walls, "Airway," in *Rosen's Emergency Medicine: Concepts and Clinical Practice,* 5th ed., ed.-in-chief J. A. Marx (Mosby, 2002).

- Assemble drugs and equipment (e.g., suction, pulse oximetry, ET tube of desired size plus tubes one size larger and smaller, stylet, bag-valve device, oropharyngeal and nasal airways, alternate airways, $ETCO_2$ detector device).
- Establish vascular access.
- Apply a cardiac monitor.

2. **P**reoxygenation (zero minus 5 minutes):
   - 100% oxygen by mask for 5 minutes or ventilate gently

3. **P**retreatment as indicated (zero minus 3 minutes):
   - Lidocaine—reduces increased intracranial pressure (ICP) response to laryngoscopy and prevents bronchospasm
   - Atropine—diminishes bradycardic response from laryngoscopic stimulation of vagus nerve
   - Defasciculation adjunct if using succinylcholine
   - Fentanyl—diminishes sympathetic response (increased heart rate and blood pressure) to laryngoscopy and intubation

4. **P**aralysis with induction (zero point):
   - Induction agent IVP
     - Thiopental, methohexital, fentanyl, ketamine, etomidate, or propofol
   - Neuromuscular blocking agent IVP

5. **P**rotection (zero + 30 seconds):
   - Apply cricoid pressure.
   - Position the patient for intubation.
   - To avoid gastric distension, do not ventilate with a bag-mask unless SpO_2 is <90%.

6. **P**lacement of tube (zero + 45 seconds):
   - Check the mandible for flaccidity.
   - Intubate, remove the stylet, and inflate the cuff.
   - Confirm tube placement.
     - Use clinical methods and confirmation devices.
   - Release cricoid pressure.

7. **P**ost-intubation management (zero + 2 minutes):
   - Secure the tube.
   - Obtain a chest X-ray.
   - Maintain long-acting sedation/paralysis.
   - Initiate mechanical ventilation.

RSI Medications

When performing rapid sequence intubation, carefully select the proper drugs to use for each step of the procedure (Table 10-1). You will need an agent for pretreatment and paralysis.

TABLE 10-1 Medications for Rapid Sequence Intubation

Agent	Purpose	IVP Dosage	Onset	Duration
Atropine	Blunts bradycardia	0.02 mg/kg	30 seconds	30 minutes
Lidocaine	Blunts laryngospasm	1–2 mg/kg	30 seconds	30 minutes
Etomidate	Sedative/induction	0.2–0.6 mg/kg	60 seconds	3–5 minutes
Fentanyl	Induction Sedation	2–10 mcg/kg 3 mcg/kg	60 seconds	30–60 minutes
Ketamine	Induction	2 mg/kg	30–60 seconds	15 minutes
Midazolam	Induction Sedation	0.07–0.30 mg/kg 0.02–0.04 mg/kg	2 minutes	1–2 hours
Propofol		2.0–2.5 mg/kg	40 seconds	3–5 minutes
Thiopental	Sedative/induction	3–5 mg/kg	20–40 seconds	5–10 minutes
Succinylcholine	Paralysis	1–2 mg/kg	30–60 seconds	4–6 minutes
Rocuronium	Paralysis	RSI: 0.60–1.20 mg/kg	2 minutes	30 minutes
Vecuronium	Paralysis	RSI: 0.1–0.2 mg/kg M: 0.1 mg/kg	2–5 minutes	30–60 minutes

RSI = intubation dose, M = maintenance dose

Pretreatment

These drugs are intended to relax the patient and lower the patient's intracranial pressure. They are referred to as sedatives and induction agents, and should be administered before the paralytic agent. Succinylcholine causes an initial short period of muscle contractions (fasciculations) before the paralytic effect occurs. This fasciculation may increase the intracranial pressure. Therefore, administration of a small dose of a nonfasciculating paralytic agent will prevent the fasciculation without producing prolonged paralysis.

Paralytic Agents

Paralytic agents are divided into two classes:

1. Depolarizing agents, such as succinylcholine
   - Cause a short period of muscle fasciculation when they depolarize the neuromuscular junction
   - Duration of action is short

- If you are unable to intubate the patient, ventilate with the BVM until the drug wears off.
2. Nondepolarizing agents
   - Do not cause muscle fasciculation
   - Have a long duration of effect
   - Administer once intubation has been confirmed and to maintain paralysis.

 # Hypothermia

Unintentional hypothermia causes generalized depression of body functions. Care for all hypothermic patients should be directed at raising the core body temperature. If the patient is not yet in arrest, handle the patient gently to avoid triggering ventricular fibrillation.

Signs and Symptoms

The progression of the signs and symptoms of hypothermia varies (Table 10-2). It depends on the ambient temperature, the preexisting physical and medical condition of the patient, and whether wind or water immersion is involved.

TABLE 10-2   Signs and Symptoms of Hypothermia

Classification	Core Body Temperature	Signs and Symptoms
Mild hypothermia	34–36°C 93.2–96.8°F	■ Increased muscle tone followed by shivering ■ Amnesia, dysarthria, ataxia
Moderate hypothermia	30–<34°C 86–<93.2°F	■ Shivering that decreases then stops ■ Oxygen consumption that slows ■ Atrial fibrillation ■ Decreasing level of consciousness
Severe hypothermia	<30°C <86°F	■ Hypotension and bradycardia ■ Usually complete unconsciousness ■ Loss of corneal and deep tendon reflexes ■ Pulmonary edema ■ High risk for ventricular fibrillation (VF) with movement ■ As temperature decreases, spontaneous VF likely ■ Progression to asystole

Hypothermia Algorithm

▶ Remove wet clothing

▶ Protect against heat loss and wind chill

↓

▶ Move to a warm environment (cover with blankets and insulating equipment)

▶ Maintain a horizontal position

▶ Handle the patient gently; avoid jostling

▶ Monitor the core temperature and cardiac rhythm

↓

▶ Assess responsiveness, breathing (assess for 30–45 seconds), and pulse (assess for 30–45 seconds)

↓

▶ If breathing and pulse present:
  - Mild hypothermia—core body temperature 34°C–36°C (93.2°–96.8°F)
    - Passive rewarming
      - Methods used may include removing wet clothes, drying the skin, and covering the body with warm blankets.
    - Active external rewarming
  - Moderate hypothermia—core body temperature 30°C–34°C (86°–93.2°F)
    - Passive rewarming
    - Active external rewarming of trunk only
      - Methods used may include electric or charcoal warming devices, hot water bottles, heating pads, radiant heat sources, and warming beds.
  - Severe hypothermia—core body temperature < 30°C (< 86°F)
    - Active internal rewarming sequence:
      - Warm IV fluids (43°C [109°F])
      - Warm, humidified O_2 (42°C–46°C [108°–115°F])
      - Peritoneal lavage (KCl-free)
      - Extracorporeal rewarming
      - Esophageal rewarming tubes
    - Continue rewarming until the core temperature is > 35°C (95°F), spontaneous circulation returns, or resuscitation efforts cease.

↓

▶ If apneic/pulseless: Cardiac arrest
  - Begin CPR
  - Defibrillate VF/pulseless VT once (120–200 J biphasic; 360 J monophasic or use AED)

- Continue CPR
- Intubate, confirm tube placement, secure the tube
- Ventilate with warm, humidified O_2 (42°C–46°C [108°–115°F])
- IV; administer warm normal saline (43°C [109°F])

▶ Assess core temperature
  - Core temperature < 30°C (86°F)
    - Continue CPR
    - Withhold IV medications until core temperature is > 30°C (86°F)
    - Limit shocks for VF/VT to one
    - Transport to the emergency department
    - Begin the active internal rewarming sequence

  - Core temperature > 30°C (86°F)
    - Continue CPR
    - Give IV meds as indicated by the algorithm, but space them at longer than standard intervals
    - Repeat defibrillation for VF/VT as the patient's core temperature rises
    - Begin the active internal rewarming sequence

 ## Drowning

Drowning is a process that causes respiratory impairment secondary to submersion or immersion in liquid.[2] See Table 10-3 for a classification of the clinical findings associated with drowning.

When caring for a drowning patient, consider that there may be a medical or traumatic cause of the episode, such as head or cervical spine trauma, drug or alcohol intoxication, seizure, hypoglycemia, hypothermia, cardiac arrest, or a cerebrovascular accident.

The two most important factors that predict patient outcome after drowning are the length of submersion and the severity of hypoxia.

Patients who need any type of resuscitation at the scene of a drowning should be transported for evaluation. Some pulmonary complications may have a delayed onset of symptoms.

---

[2] A. H. Idris et al., "ILCOR Advisory Statement: Recommended Guidelines for Uniform Reporting of Data from Drowning-The Utstsein Style," *Circulation* 108, no. 20 (Nov. 18, 2003): 2565–2574.

TABLE 10-3   Classification of Clinical Findings Associated with Submersion

Clinical Findings	Severity	Mortality
Normal pulmonary auscultation with coughing	1	0%
Abnormal pulmonary auscultation with rales in some pulmonary fields	2	0.6%
Abnormal pulmonary auscultation with rales in all pulmonary fields (acute pulmonary edema) without arterial hypotension	3	5.2%
Abnormal pulmonary auscultation with rales in all pulmonary fields (acute pulmonary edema) with arterial hypotension	4	19.4%
Isolated respiratory arrest	5	44%
Cardiopulmonary arrest	6	93%

Source: CHEST by D. SZPILMAN. Copyright 1997 by AM COLLEGE OF CHEST PHYSICIANS. Reproduced with permission of AM COLLEGE OF CHEST PHYSICIANS in the format Textbook via Copyright Clearance Center.

Interventions for the Drowning Patient

General interventions for the drowning patient include the following actions:

- Ensure scene and rescuer safety.
- Assess the victim's airway, breathing, and pulse.
- If a cervical spine injury is suspected, stabilize the victim's head and neck in a neutral position and, if indicated, open the airway using a jaw thrust without head tilt.
- If indicated, provide rescue breathing as soon as is safely possible.
- After delivering 2 rescue breaths, check for signs of circulation for 10 seconds.
- If no pulse is detected, begin chest compressions. (Note that a pulse may be difficult to palpate due to peripheral vasoconstriction).
  - Chest compressions may be attempted in the water by trained rescuers.
- Dry the patient's chest and attach an AED, if available. (Ensure patient and rescuer safety before delivering shocks.) If indicated, deliver one shock; resume CPR and then assess the patient's core body temperature.
- If the patient's core body temperature is < 30°C (< 86°F), follow the hypothermia algorithm.
- If these efforts are unsuccessful, resume BLS and ACLS care.
- Maintain the patient's body temperature. Dry and warm the victim.
- Do not attempt to drain water from the patient's lungs.

ACLS Management

Other Advanced Cardiac Life Support interventions to consider when caring for a patient who has drowned include the following:

- Intubating apneic or unresponsive patients
  - Improves oxygenation and ventilation
  - Reduces risk of aspiration
  - Allows direct removal of foreign material from the airway
  - Allows application of continuous positive airway pressure (CPAP) or positive end-expiratory pressure (PEEP)
- Establishing vascular access
- Managing hypothermia, if present
- Transporting the patient to a hospital for further evaluation and treatment if any rescue measure was needed

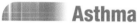 **Asthma**

Severe asthma accounts for many deaths and admissions to intensive care units annually.[3]

Pathophysiology

The signs and symptoms of asthma are related to three problems:

1. Bronchoconstriction
2. Inflammation of the small airways
3. Excessive mucus

Asthma severity can be mild, moderate, or severe. Treatment decisions are made based on severity.

Near-Fatal Asthma

Near-fatal asthma is identified by respiratory arrest or evidence of respiratory failure ($PaCO_2 > 50$ mmHg). There are two types:

1. Slow-onset, near-fatal asthma
   - The gradual progression of asthma symptoms occurs over several days.
2. Rapid-onset, near-fatal asthma
   - Symptom onset and progression to a life-threatening condition occur in ≤ 3 hours.

Risk Factors for Death from Asthma

The following risk factors are associated with an increased risk of fatal or near-fatal asthma attacks:

- Past history of sudden, severe asthma attacks

---

[3] National Institutes of Health, National Heart, Lung, and Blood Institute, *Guidelines for the Diagnosis and Management of Asthma,* NIH Publication No. 97-4051 (July 1977).

- Prior intubation for asthma
- Admission to an intensive care unit for asthma in the past
- Recent hospitalization for asthma
- Dependency on steroids or recent withdrawal from oral steroids
- Other serious cardiac or pulmonary disease
- Serious psychiatric disease, including depression or anxiety
- Street drug use, especially inhaled cocaine and heroin
- Poor perception of asthma severity
- Environmental exposures (inner-city residents, air pollution, cigarette smoking)
- African American males
- Patients who wait to seek care
- Patients who don't notify their physician of worsening symptoms
- Patients who were diagnosed with asthma before the age of 5

Possible Presentations[4]

The National Heart, Lung, and Blood Institute and World Health Organization describe the assessment parameters below to help distinguish asthma severity.

Mild Asthma[5]

- Breathless when walking; can lie down
- Talks in sentences
- May be agitated
- Respiratory rate increased
- Moderate wheezing, often only on end-expiration
- Heart rate < 100 bpm
- *Pulsus paradoxus* usually absent
- Peek expiratory flow (PEF) after initial bronchodilator $> 80\%$ predicted or personal best
- PaO_2 (on room air) normal
- $PaCO_2 < 45$ mmHg

Figure 10-1 depicts mild asthma.

Moderate Asthma[6]

- Breathless when talking; prefers sitting
- Talks in phrases

---

[4] Ibid.
[5] Ibid.
[6] Ibid.

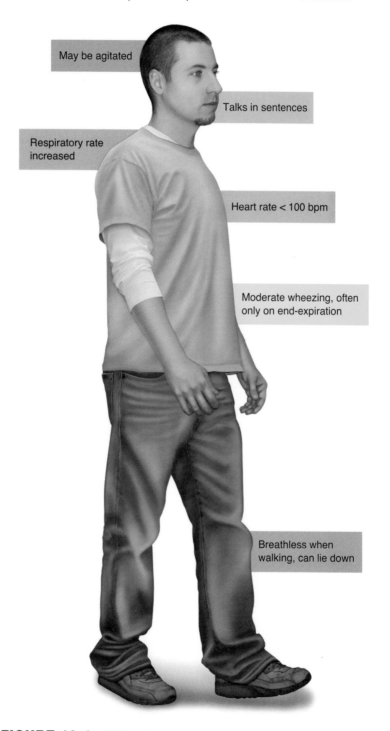

FIGURE 10-1   Mild asthma.

- Usually agitated
- Respiratory rate increased
- Accessory muscle use and suprasternal retractions usually present
- Loud wheezing
- Heart rate 100–120 bpm
- *Pulsus paradoxus* may be present
- PEF after initial bronchodilator approximately 60–80% predicted or personal best
- PaO_2 (on room air) > 60 mmHg
- $PaCO_2 > 45$ mmHg
- SaO_2 91–95%

Severe Asthma[7]

- Breathless at rest; hunched forward
- Talks in single words or is too breathless to speak
- Usually agitated
- Respiratory rate often > 30 breaths/minute
- Accessory muscle use and suprasternal retractions usually present
- Usually loud wheezing
- Heart rate > 120 bpm
- *Pulsus paradoxus* often present
- PEF after initial bronchodilator approximately $< 60\%$ predicted or personal best (< 100 L/min in adults)
- PaO_2 (on room air) < 60 mmHg; possible cyanosis
- $PaCO_2 > 45$ mmHg; possible respiratory failure
- $SaO_2 < 90\%$

Figure 10-2 depicts severe asthma.

Imminent Respiratory Arrest[8]

Imminent respiratory arrest is characterized by the following:

- Markedly decreased level of consciousness
- Paradoxical thoracoabdominal movement
- Bradycardia
- Absence of wheezing (silent chest)
- Absence of *pulsus paradoxus* suggests respiratory muscle fatigue

---

[7] Ibid.
[8] Ibid.

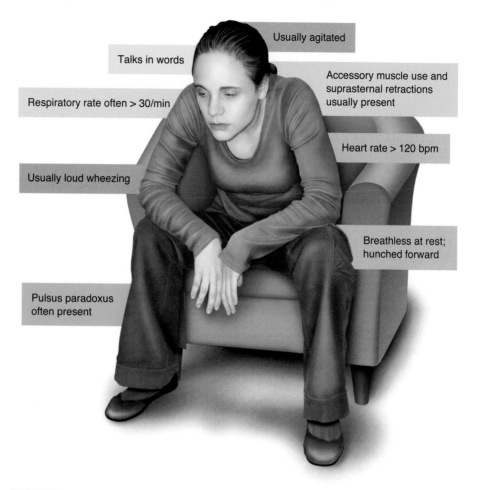

Usually agitated

Talks in words

Accessory muscle use and suprasternal retractions usually present

Respiratory rate often > 30/min

Heart rate > 120 bpm

Usually loud wheezing

Breathless at rest; hunched forward

Pulsus paradoxus often present

FIGURE 10-2   Severe asthma.

Possible Interventions[9]

The following information from the National Institutes of Health provides assessment and treatment guidelines for asthma:

- Initial assessment
  - History
  - Physical examination
    - Auscultation
    - Use of accessory muscles
    - Heart rate

[9] Ibid.

- Respiratory rate
- PEF or FEV$_1$ (forced expiratory volume in 1 second)
- Oxygen saturation
- Arterial blood gas of patient in extremis
- Other tests as indicated

Note: Preferred treatments are inhaled beta-2 agonists such as albuterol (or levalbuterol), anticholinergic agents such as atrovent, and steroids. If inhaled beta-2 agonists are not available, methylxanthines may be considered.

- Initial treatment
  - Inhaled rapid-acting beta-2 agonist, usually by nebulization, one dose every 20 minutes for 1 hour
  - Oxygen to achieve O$_2$ saturation $\geq$ 90% in adults
  - Systemic steroids (methylprednisolone) if no immediate response, patient recently took an oral steroid, or if the episode is severe
  - Sedation is contraindicated.
- Repeat assessment
  - Physical examination, PEF, O$_2$ saturation
- Moderate episode
  - Treatment
    - Administer inhaled beta-2 agonist and inhaled anticholinergic agents by nebulization.
    - If failure to respond to inhaled beta-2 agonist within 1 hour, consider placing patient on continuously inhaled beta-2 agonist for 1–3 hours.
    - Consider administration of epinephrine or terbutaline subcutaneously.
    - Consider use of BiPAP ventilatory support.
    - Consider steroids.
    - Continue treatment 1–3 hours, provided there is improvement.
- Severe episode
  - Signs and symptoms
    - PEF < 60% of predicted/personal best
    - Physical exam: severe symptoms at rest, chest retractions
    - Hx: high-risk patient
    - No improvement after the initial treatment
  - Treatment
    - Administer inhaled beta-2 agonist and inhaled anticholinergic via continuous nebulization.
    - Provide oxygen.
    - Administer systemic steroids via IV.
    - Administer SC, IM, or IV beta-2 agonist.
    - Institute BiPAP ventilatory support.

- Consider IV methylxanthines.
- Consider IV magnesium.

Intubation and Ventilation in Status Asthmaticus

When intubation of the severe asthmatic is needed, rapid sequence intubation is preferred. The patient should be intubated using the largest ET tube possible to minimize airway resistance during ventilation.

When delivering positive-pressure ventilation to patients in status asthmaticus, breath stacking can cause hyperinflation of the lungs. This may lead to tension pneumothorax and hypotension. To minimize the risk of these complications:

- Sedate the patient.
- Continue nebulized bronchodilator treatments.
- Ventilate at 6–10 breaths/minute.
- Reduce the tidal volume to 6–8 mL/kg.
- Deliver breaths using a shorter inspiratory time and a longer expiratory time:
  - Inspiratory to expiratory ratios of 1:4 or 1:5

If the intubated asthma patient deteriorates suddenly, the patient should be immediately assessed for airway complications.

- Reevaluate for correct tube placement.
- Suction the patient to detect any obstructions in the ET tube.
- Assess for tension pneumothorax.
- Check the equipment to ensure that the correct amount of oxygen is being delivered and that there are no malfunctions.

◆ ◇ ◇ **Testing Tips**

- Remember the DOPE mnemonic and check for the following: tube **D**isplacement or **O**bstruction, **P**neumothorax, or **E**quipment failure.

Anaphylaxis

Anaphylaxis is a severe, life-threatening, systemic allergic reaction. It manifests with serious signs and symptoms that affect two or more body systems.

Signs and Symptoms

Of all of the signs and symptoms of anaphylaxis, the cutaneous indicators are the ones that most frequently help the provider to distinguish anaphylaxis from other medical conditions. The clinical effects of anaphylaxis can be divided by body system (Table 10-4). The signs and symptoms of anaphylaxis are illustrated in Figure 10-3.

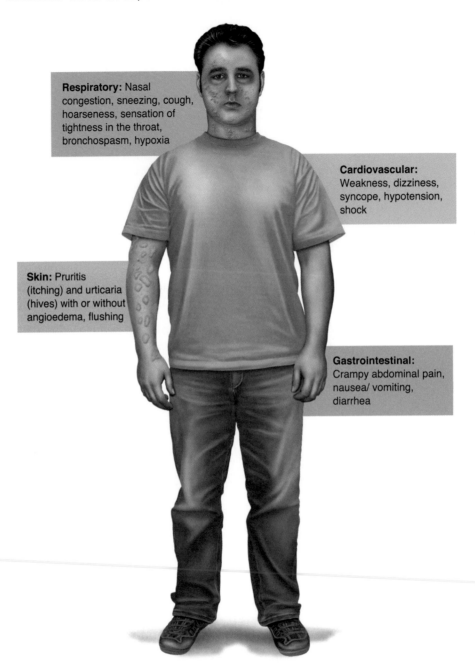

Respiratory: Nasal congestion, sneezing, cough, hoarseness, sensation of tightness in the throat, bronchospasm, hypoxia

Cardiovascular: Weakness, dizziness, syncope, hypotension, shock

Skin: Pruritis (itching) and urticaria (hives) with or without angioedema, flushing

Gastrointestinal: Crampy abdominal pain, nausea/ vomiting, diarrhea

FIGURE 10-3 The signs and symptoms of anaphylaxis.

TABLE 10-4 Clinical Effects of Anaphylaxis

Body System	Anaphylactic Effects
Respiratory	Upper airway swelling: ■ Hoarseness ■ Difficulty swallowing ■ Stridor ■ Complete airway obstruction Lower airway effects: ■ Bronchospasm ■ Wheezing ■ Dyspnea
Cardiovascular	Cardiovascular collapse related to hypovolemia: ■ Absolute hypovolemia from capillary leak ■ Relative hypovolemia from vasodilation
Cutaneous	Urticaria Angioedema Pruritis Erythema
Gastrointestinal	Abdominal pain Vomiting and diarrhea

Differential Diagnosis

It is important to distinguish anaphylaxis from other conditions that present with similar signs and symptoms. Failure to do so can result in death of the patient. Some of these conditions are:

- Angioedema related to ACE inhibitor treatment
- Asthma-induced bronchospasm
- Food aspiration
- Hereditary angioedema
  - Patient does not respond to standard anaphylaxis management
  - Patient must be given fresh frozen plasma or C1 esterase inhibitor
- Scombroid poisoning
  - Spoiled fish
- Panic disorder with stridor
- Septic shock
- Upper airway obstruction
- Vasovagal reactions

Possible Interventions

Manage anaphylaxis rapidly and aggressively to prevent airway obstruction and cardiovascular collapse.

- Administer high-concentration oxygen.
  - Assist ventilations with a bag-valve-mask device, if necessary.
  - Bag-valve-mask ventilation and tracheal intubation may be impossible due to alteration of the airway anatomy by edema. Consult with an anesthesiologist or an ENT specialist if rapidly accessible.
  - Consider intubation in the presence of:
    - Hoarseness
    - Swelling of the tongue
    - Stridor
    - Swelling in the oropharynx
    - Severe angioedema
  - Surgical airway intervention using standard cricothyrotomy may be necessary but impossible due to obliteration of landmarks by severe swelling. Consider:
    - Fiberoptic tracheal intubation
    - Digital tracheal intubation with a small tracheal tube (< 7 mm)
    - Needle cricothyrotomy with transtracheal oxygenation
- Apply cardiac monitor
- Establish large-caliber IV and administer normal saline or Ringer's lactate.
  - Infuse at TKO rate if vital signs are stable and signs/symptoms are limited to cutaneous manifestations.
  - If hypotension or tachycardia is present, administer a fluid bolus of 1–2 L for adults.
    - Additional fluid therapy should be guided by the patient's response.
    - Monitor the patient closely for the development of pulmonary edema.
- Administer epinephrine to patients with airway edema, marked respiratory distress, or signs of shock.
  - In severe anaphylaxis with an immediate life threat, administer epinephrine 0.1 mg (1:10,000) IVP over 5 minutes.
  - In moderate anaphylaxis or if vascular access has not yet been established, administer epinephrine 0.3–0.5 mg (1:1000) IM. Repeat in 15–20 minutes if no improvement.
- Administer diphenhydramine 10–50 mg slow IVP or deep IM.
- Administer histamine-2 (H_2) antagonist (e.g., cimetidine 300 mg PO, IM, or IV).
- Treat bronchospasm with an inhaled beta-2 agonist (e.g., albuterol, levalbuterol) after epinephrine is given.
  - Inhaled ipratropium may be useful for treatment of bronchospasm in patients taking beta-blockers.

- Corticosteroids are used to reduce the incidence and severity of delayed reactions.
  - Consider the use of methylprednisolone sodium succinate 125 mg IVP.
- Glucagon 1–2 mg IM or IVP may be effective for patients unresponsive to epinephrine and may be particularly useful for patients taking beta-blockers.

Interventions in Cardiac Arrest

Most of the recommendations for the management of cardiac arrest secondary to anaphylaxis are based on low-level consensus agreement rather than high-level evidence. Recommendations from the American Heart Association include the following:[10]

- Standard care for pulseless arrest
- Administer large volumes of crystalloid fluids (4–8 liters).
- Give epinephrine in escalating doses.
- Prolonged resuscitation may be needed.

 # Cardiac Arrest Associated with Trauma

Survival from cardiac arrest caused by traumatic injury is largely related to the mechanism of injury (blunt versus penetrating trauma), the age and preexisting health of the patient, and the time until the patient receives definitive care.

Overview

Survival after blunt, traumatic cardiopulmonary arrest is rare, even with maximal resuscitative efforts, mainly because the arrest may be secondary to causes that are difficult to reverse rapidly (e.g., brain injury, high spinal cord injury, proximal aortic disruption, and exsanguination from injuries).

Cardiac arrest due to penetrating trauma, particularly to the thorax, has a better prognosis than blunt or multisystem penetrating trauma. The best survival rates are in patients with stab wounds to the heart in whom cardiac arrest is attributable to cardiac tamponade. Perform pericardiocentesis on these patients for temporary stabilization until surgical repair can be accomplished.

If the patient has sinus rhythm and nondilated reactive pupils, survival may be more likely.[11]

Possible Interventions

Many actions must be performed quickly in the care of the critically injured patient. Rapid transport to a facility with definitive care should be a high priority.

---

[10] American Heart Association, "AHA Guidelines for Cardiopulmonary Resuscitation and Emergency Cardiovascular Care," *Circulation* 112, suppl. 1 (2005): IV-145.

[11] S. M. Cera, G. Mostafa, R. F. Sing, J. L. Sarafin, B. D. Matthews, and B. T. Heniford, "Physiologic Predictors of Survival in Post-Traumatic Arrest," *Am. Surg.* 69, no. 2 (Feb 2003): 140–144. PMID: 12641355.

Primary Survey

- Airway/C-Spine
  - Open the airway with a jaw-thrust without head-tilt maneuver if head, neck, or multisystem trauma is present or suspected.
    - If you are unable to open the airway with this maneuver, use the head tilt–chin lift maneuver.
  - Use a second rescuer to maintain in-line spinal immobilization until a cervical collar is applied and the patient is properly secured to a long spine board.
  - Suction the mouth of blood, vomitus, or other secretions if needed.
  - Insert an oropharyngeal airway.
- Breathing
  - Ventilate with a bag-valve-mask device or mouth-to-barrier device.
  - Seal any open chest wounds with an occlusive dressing taped on three sides.
    - If a tension pneumothorax develops after sealing an open pneumothorax, lift one corner of the occlusive dressing.
- Circulation
  - If you are unable to palpate a carotid pulse, begin chest compressions.
- Defibrillation if necessary
  - Apply the AED or manual defibrillator. If ventricular fibrillation or ventricular tachycardia is present, defibrillate once.
    - Resume CPR immediately.

Secondary Survey

- Airway
  - Perform tracheal intubation if indicated. Confirm tube placement using clinical and mechanical methods and secure the tube.
    - Cricothyrotomy is indicated if tracheal intubation is unsuccessful and you are unable to ventilate the patient.
      - This may occur if massive facial injury and edema are present.
  - Insert a gastric tube to decompress the stomach. Confirm tube placement.
- Breathing
  - Auscultate the chest bilaterally.
  - Suspect a flail chest if paradoxical movement of the chest is present.
    - If a significant flail chest is present, intubate the trachea and ventilate with positive-pressure ventilation.
  - If shock and severe respiratory distress are present, assume a tension pneumothorax if breath sounds are decreased or absent on one side and chest expansion is inadequate with positive-pressure ventilation.
    - Other late signs of tension pneumothorax include jugular venous distension and tracheal deviation away from the pneumothorax.
    - Perform needle decompression in the second or third intercostal space in the midclavicular line on the affected side. Then insert a chest tube.

- Circulation
    - Continue cardiac monitoring.
    - Stop obvious uncontrolled external bleeding.
    - Establish two large-bore IVs of normal saline or lactated ringers.
        - Fluid volume replacement is guided by the patient's blood pressure, the nature of the injury (blunt versus penetrating), and the distance to definitive care (surgery if indicated).
    - Prehospital providers should establish IVs and give medications en route to the hospital.
    - Manage arrhythmias per the appropriate algorithm.
        - PEA and bradyasystolic rhythms are the most common terminal cardiac rhythms observed in trauma victims, as they are consistent with hypovolemic shock. Initiate aggressive fluid administration and consider the use of vasopressors.
        - It is vital to address the underlying cause and treat it!
- Differential diagnosis
    - Consider possible nontraumatic causes of the arrest (hypothermia, hypoglycemia, overdose, underlying medical conditions, etc.).
- Consider open thoracotomy (especially if penetrating chest trauma) if the patient arrested:
    - Immediately prior to arrival at the ED
    - After arrival at the ED

Guidelines for Withholding or Terminating Resuscitation in Prehospital Traumatic Cardiopulmonary Arrest[12]

Note: These recommendations do not address the following groups of patients: (1) pediatric patients, (2) patients in whom a medical cause (such as myocardial infarction) precipitated the arrest, and (3) patients with complicating factors, such as the potential for severe hypothermia.

- Blunt traumatic cardiopulmonary arrest
    - Resuscitation efforts may be withheld if, after a thorough primary assessment, the patient is found apneic, pulseless, and without organized ECG activity upon EMS arrival.
- Penetrating traumatic cardiopulmonary arrest
    - Begin resuscitation if the patient is found apneic and pulseless by EMS, but other signs of life (e.g., pupillary reflexes, spontaneous movement, or organized ECG activity) are present.

---

[12] L. R. Hopson et al., National Association of EMS Physicians Standards and Clinical Practice Committee, American College of Surgeons Committee on Trauma, "Guidelines for Withholding or Termination of Resuscitation in Prehospital Traumatic Cardiopulmonary Arrest: A Joint Position Paper from the National Association of EMS Physicians Standards and Clinical Practice Committee and the American College of Surgeons Committee on Trauma," *Prehosp. Emerg. Care* 7, no. 1 (Jan.–Mar. 2003): 141–146. PMID: 12540158.

- Transport to the nearest emergency department or trauma center.
- Resuscitation efforts may be withheld if these signs of life are absent.
- Blunt or penetrating traumatic cardiopulmonary arrest
  - Begin resuscitation efforts in cardiac arrest patients in whom the mechanism of injury does not correlate with their clinical condition, suggesting a nontraumatic cause of the arrest.
  - Consider termination of efforts in the following patients:
    - Trauma patients with EMS-witnessed cardiopulmonary arrest and 15 minutes of unsuccessful resuscitation and CPR
    - Traumatic cardiopulmonary arrest patients with a transport time to an ED or trauma center of more than 15 minutes after the arrest is identified (considered nonsalvageable)
  - Do not begin resuscitation if:
    - There is evidence of a significant time lapse since pulselessness (e.g., dependent lividity, rigor mortis, decomposition).
    - Injuries are obviously incompatible with life (e.g., decapitation, hemicorporectomy).
- Give special consideration to victims of drowning and lightning strikes and in situations in which significant hypothermia may alter the patient's prognosis.

Cardiac Arrest Associated with Pregnancy

Although cardiac arrest in pregnancy is uncommon, it presents unique challenges because of the physiologic changes associated with pregnancy, and also because two lives are at risk.

Causes of Maternal Cardiac Arrest

The causes of maternal cardiac arrest include the following:

- Trauma (e.g., motor vehicle crashes, assaults, falls)
- Pulmonary embolism
- Congenital or acquired cardiac disease
- Hemorrhage
- Hypoxia
- Hypotension
- Drug overdose
- Sepsis
- Pregnancy-induced hypertension (PIH)
- Congestive cardiomyopathy
- Aortic dissection
- Amniotic fluid embolism
- Sickle cell disease

- Complications of tocolytic therapy
- Complications of epidural analgesia
- Drug toxicity or hypersensitivity
- Water intoxication

Physiological Changes During Pregnancy—Implications for Maternal Resuscitation

Some techniques in maternal resuscitation may need to be modified based on the physiologic changes during the third trimester of pregnancy. Some of these changes also place the pregnant female at risk of cardiac arrest in certain situations.

Pulmonary System

- Reduced functional residual capacity (FRC) because the gravid uterus elevates the diaphragm
- Oxygen demand increased 20% due to pregnancy; decreased cardiopulmonary reserve
- Tension pneumothorax may develop more quickly in pregnancy due to diaphragm elevation and pulmonary hyperventilation.

Cardiovascular System

- Expanded blood volume
- Vasodilation occurs due to progesterone
- Signs of maternal hypotension from acute traumatic bleeding may be delayed. Fetal compromise can be far advanced by the time obvious signs of shock appear in the mother.
- Increased risk of thromboembolism
- Aortocaval compression (Figures 10-4 and 10-5)

Gastrointestinal System

- Delayed gastric emptying
- Relaxation of the lower esophageal sphincter due to the influence of progesterone
- Commonly, passive reflux of gastric contents
- Increased risk of aspiration

Maternal Resuscitation

When resuscitating a pregnant woman, use the ACLS algorithms without modifying medications, intubation, and defibrillation. Displace the uterus to the left throughout the resuscitative efforts.

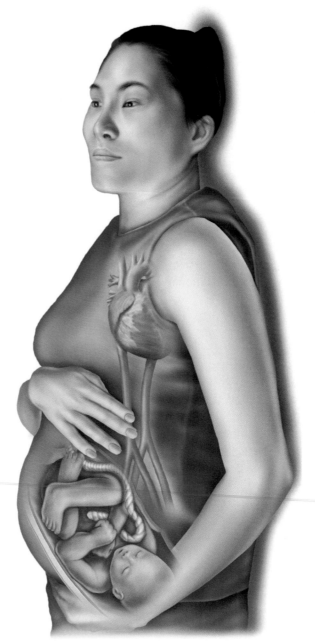

FIGURE 10-4 Aortocaval compression. After approximately the 20th week of gestation, the gravid uterus compresses the inferior vena cava and abdominal aorta when the patient is supine. This decreases cardiac preload, cardiac output, and uterine blood flow.

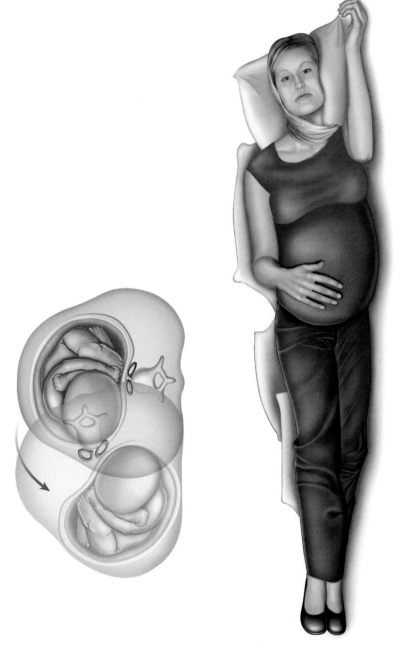

FIGURE 10-5 Relieving pressure on the abdominal vessels during pregnancy. Place the pregnant patient in the left lateral position or manually displace the uterus to the left to move the gravid uterus off the abdominal vessels.

If the possibility of fetal viability exists, a perimortem cesarean delivery should be performed within 5 minutes of maternal cardiac arrest in order to maximize the chances of maternal and infant survival. This should be performed only in the hospital setting.

Electric Shock and Lightning Strikes

Lightning or electric current passing through the body causes electric shock injuries. Nerve and blood vessel tissues are low resistors to electrical energy. Therefore, when the current entry/exit path is from hand to hand, the current often passes through the heart and can cause ventricular fibrillation.

Factors That Determine the Severity of Injury

The severity of electrical burn injury is related to voltage, amperage, current type, length of current exposure, and the pathway of the current through the body:

- The current's pressure (voltage)
  - The severity of injury due to electric shock is determined largely by current voltage. Low voltage is 1000 volts or less. High voltage is more than 1000 volts.
  - In some situations, low voltage can be as harmful as high voltage.
- The amount of current (amperage)
  - 1 ampere is approximately equal to the amount of current passing through a 100-watt light bulb.
  - VF can occur at 50–120 milliamperes (mA).
- The type of current (direct vs. alternating)
  - Contact with high-voltage direct current often throws the victim from the source. Blunt trauma is possible if the patient falls.
  - Contact with alternating current can cause tetanic muscle contractions that "freeze" the patient to the current source. This increases the duration of exposure to the electrical energy and increases injury severity.
    - The frequent pulses from alternating current also make it more likely that the current will stimulate the heart during the relative refractory period, creating an "R on T" phenomenon that causes ventricular fibrillation.
  - Lightning is neither a direct current nor an alternating current. Lightning is a current phenomenon, rather than a voltage phenomenon.[13]
- Body tissue resistance to the current varies greatly.
  - Muscles, nerves, and blood vessels have the least resistance to current because of their high electrolyte and water content.
  - Bones, tendons, and fat have a very high resistance to current.
  - Skin resistance depends on its wetness, thickness, and cleanliness. Thick or dry skin is more resistant than thin or wet skin.

---

[13] T. G. Price and M. A. Cooper, "Electrical and Lightning Injuries," in *Rosen's Emergency Medicine: Concepts and Clinical Practice,* 5th ed., ed.-in-chief J. A. Marx (Mosby, 2002).

- The current's pathway through the body
  - A hand-to-hand (transthoracic) pathway is more likely to be fatal than a hand-to-foot (vertical) or foot-to-foot (straddle) current pathway.
  - Transthoracic current flow can cause cardiac arrhythmias and direct myocardial damage. If current passes through the brain, respiratory arrest, seizures, and paralysis may result.
- Duration of contact with the current source
  - The longer the contact with the current source, the greater the likelihood of electrical injury.

Mechanisms of Injury

Primary Injury

The primary electrical injury is burns, which can be classified into two categories:

1. Direct contact
   - Electrothermal heating
2. Indirect contact
   - Arc
   - Flame
   - Flash

Secondary Injury

Secondary injury may result from a fall or being thrown from the electrical source by intense muscle contraction or secondary damage to other tissues. It includes the following:

- Fractures (cervical spine, skull, femur, humerus)
- Closed head injury
- Peripheral nerve injury
- Myoglobinuria

Emergency Care

It is critical to first consider the mechanism of injury when you provide care to a patient with an electrical injury. Consider safety, internal organ damage, and the potential for secondary injuries as you treat these patients. Your interventions should include the following:

- Ensure rescuer safety.
  - If possible, turn off the power source.
  - Removal of a patient from a live power source should be done only by rescuers who are properly equipped and trained to do so.

- Triage considerations:
    - Triage of patients struck by lightning should place the highest priority on those who are in cardiac or respiratory arrest.
    - The lightning strike victim who develops immediate cardiac arrest has a high likelihood of survival and recovery if BLS is begun immediately.
- Protect the cervical spine and treat the injuries.
- Treat VF, asystole, and other arrhythmias according to the ACLS algorithms for these rhythms.
    - Continue resuscitative efforts for a longer period than usual.
- Airway compromise is possible in patients with burns of the face, mouth, or anterior neck due to soft-tissue swelling. Consider intubation early.
- Aggressive IV fluid administration may be necessary to correct ongoing fluid losses and avoid renal failure due to myoglobinuria.
- Initiate IV access in an unburned upper extremity if possible. Avoid vascular access in an extremity with an electrical burn.

Electrolyte Disorders

Electrolyte disorders can be difficult to detect. The patient may present with vague signs or symptoms that can represent many illnesses. ACLS providers should consider past medical history, home medicines, and ECG findings to have a high-index of suspicion for these abnormalities. Confirmation is not possible in the prehospital setting—laboratory analysis of a blood specimen provides the definitive diagnosis.

Potassium

Normal serum potassium is 3.5–5.0 mEq/L. Serum potassium levels reflect *extracellular* potassium levels and do not indicate the amount of intracellular potassium.

Hyperkalemia

ECG findings in hyperkalemia are illustrated in Figure 10-6.

Causes
- The causes of hyperkalemia can include any of the following:
    - Acute or chronic kidney failure
    - Lupus nephritis
    - Kidney transplant rejection
    - Glomerulonephritis
    - Diet or medications
    - Aldosterone deficiency (e.g., Addison's disease)
    - Traumatic injury
    - Hemolytic conditions
    - Rhabdomyolysis from drug ingestion, alcoholism, or coma
    - Some infections

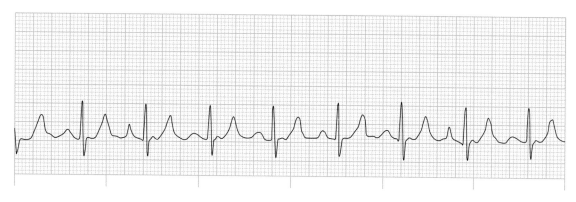

FIGURE 10-6 Hyperkalemia.

Signs and Symptoms

- Generalized fatigue, weakness, hypotension, paresthesias, palpitations, ascending paralysis, respiratory failure, bradycardia, diminished deep tendon reflexes, or decreased motor strength
- ECG changes include tall, peaked (tented) T waves (early ECG change); prolonged PR and QT intervals; flattened P waves and ST segments; widened QRS
  - Can lead to idioventricular rhythm and asystole

Treatment

- O_2, IV, monitor, vital signs
- Monitor ECG continuously or with serial ECGs
- Order lab studies:
  - Potassium
  - BUN and creatinine
  - Glucose, calcium levels
  - Digoxin level if the patient is taking a digitalis preparation
  - Arterial blood gases (ABG) if suspected pH disturbance
  - Urinalysis
- Mild hyperkalemia (5–6 mEq/L)
  - Treatment goal is to remove potassium with one or more of the following:
    - Furosemide 40–80 mg slow IVP
    - Kayexalate 15–30 g in 50–100 mL of 20% sorbitol (orally or via retention enema) to bind potassium and eliminate it from the GI tract
- Moderate hyperkalemia (6.0–7.0 mEq/L). Use measures above and:
  - Temporarily shift potassium into the cells by using one of the following:
    - Glucose and insulin: Give 10 U regular insulin IV plus 25 g (50 mL) of $D_{50}W$ over 15–30 minutes
    - Nebulized albuterol 10–20 mg over 15 minutes
    - Sodium bicarbonate 50 mEq IVP over 5 minutes

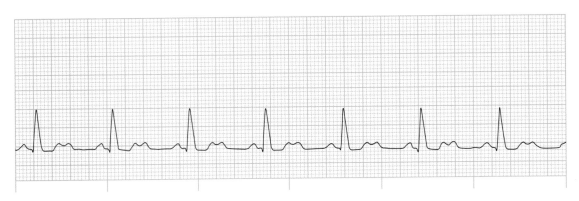

FIGURE 10-7   Hypokalemia.

- Severe hyperkalemia (> 7 mEq/L) Use measures noted earlier and:
  - Give calcium chloride 500 mg to 1 g (5–10 mL) of 10% solution slow IVP over 2–5 minutes to counteract the muscular and cardiac effects of hyperkalemia, including cardiac arrhythmias.
  - Temporarily shift potassium into the cells as for moderate hyperkalemia.
  - Remove potassium from the body as for mild hyperkalemia.

Hypokalemia

Hypokalemia is a potassium level < 3.5 mEq/L. ECG findings in hypokalemia are illustrated in Figure 10-7.

Causes

- The causes of hypokalemia can include any of the following:
  - Malnutrition
  - Increased excretion of potassium due to the prolonged use of potassium depleting diuretics (common cause)
  - Gastric suctioning, vomiting, or diarrhea or laxative use
  - Severe hyperglycemia
  - Antibiotic use (carbenicillin, sodium penicillin, amphotericin B)
  - Renal loss from hyperaldosteronism

Signs and Symptoms

- The signs and symptoms of hypokalemia affect many body systems, but the most significant clinical effects relate to the cardiac nerves and muscles.
  - Nervous system
    - Psychosis, delirium, or hallucinations
    - Depression

- Musculoskeletal
  - Skeletal muscle weakness or cramps
  - Fasciculations or tetany
  - Decreased deep tendon reflexes
  - Paralysis, or paresthesias
- Gastrointestinal
  - Constipation, ileus, nausea/vomiting, abdominal cramps
- Renal
  - Polyuria, nocturia, or polydipsia,
- Cardiovascular
  - Palpitations
  - Hypotension
  - Atrial arrhythmias
  - Early ECG changes include flattening or inversion of the T wave, a prominent U wave, and ST-segment depression
  - Severe hypokalemia may result in a prolonged PR interval, decreased voltage and widening of the QRS complex, and an increased risk of ventricular arrhythmias.
  - Cardiac arrest

Treatment

- O_2, IV, monitor, vital signs
- Monitor ECG continuously or with serial ECGs
- Order lab studies:
  - Potassium
  - BUN and creatinine
  - Glucose, magnesium, calcium, and/or phosphorous if other electrolyte disturbances are suspected
  - Digoxin level if the patient is taking a digitalis preparation
  - ABGs if suspected pH disturbance
- Moderate hypokalemia (2.5–3.0 mEq/L)
  - Oral potassium replacement therapy is preferable to IV therapy because the risk of hyperkalemia is significantly less.
  - IV potassium replacement therapy is typically reserved for patients who cannot tolerate oral replacement therapy, with serious symptoms (e.g., arrhythmias), and with severe hypokalemia.
- Severe hypokalemia ($<$ 2.5 mEq/L)
  - IV potassium replacement at a rate of 10–20 mEq/hr diluted appropriately.
    - Monitor ECG during infusion
    - Use a central line for potassium concentrations exceeding 20 mEq/L. Because the infusion of potassium into the coronary sinus may contribute to life-threatening arrhythmias, ensure that the tip of the central line catheter is not positioned in the right atrium.

Sodium

The normal sodium range is 135–145 mEq/L. Normal sodium levels are important to help regulate fluid balance. When sodium levels increase, serum osmolality increases, and when sodium levels decrease, osmolality decreases. The body's levels of sodium and water are closely linked. A change in one often affects the other.

Hypernatremia

Hypernatremia is a serum sodium concentration > 145 mEq/L.

Causes

- The causes of hypokalemia can include any of the following:
  - Normovolemic hypernatremia
    - Increased insensible loss (e.g., Kussmaul respirations, tachypnea)
    - Diabetes insipidus
    - Isotonic fluid replacement of hypotonic losses
  - Hypovolemic hypernatremia
    - Decreased water intake
    - Impaired thirst mechanism
    - Diuretics (e.g., loop, thiazide, and potassium-sparing diuretics)
    - Diabetes insipidus
    - Renal losses (osmotic diuresis by means of glucose, urea, Mannitol)
    - Insensible losses through sweating, fever, respiration
    - GI losses (e.g., nasogastric suction, vomiting, diarrhea)
    - Severe burn injury
  - Hypervolemic hypernatremia
    - Excessive sodium bicarbonate therapy
    - Excessive IV hypertonic saline
    - Mineralcorticoid excess (e.g., Cushing's syndrome, Conn's syndrome, therapeutic steroid administration, excessive licorice ingestion, chewing tobacco)
    - Excessive sodium ingestion (e.g., salt tablet ingestion, sea water ingestion or drowning, bleach ingestion)

Signs and Symptoms

- The serum sodium level is often 150 mEq/L or more before symptoms are observed. Signs and symptoms are primarily CNS related due to the effects of fluid shifts on brain cells (e.g., lethargy, confusion, weakness, irritability, ataxia, hyperreflexia, tremor, seizures, and coma).
- Hypovolemic hypernatremia
  - Weight loss, decreased skin turgor, dry mucous membranes, furrowed tongue, flat neck veins, tachycardia, cool extremities
- Hypervolemic hypernatremia

- Weight gain, distended neck veins, peripheral edema, pulmonary crackles, increased central venous pressure

Treatment

- O$_2$, IV, monitor, vital signs
- Calculate water deficit:
  - Water deficit (in L) =

    $$\frac{([NA^+]_{measured} - 140)}{140} \times TBW$$

    - TBW (total body water)
      - $TBW_{in\ L} = (0.6_{men}$ or $0.5_{women}) \times Weight_{kg}$
      - A factor of 0.6 represents the normal proportion of body weight that is water. A factor of 0.5 should be used for young women and elderly men. A factor of 0.4 should be used for elderly women.
    - Weight is current body weight (kg); Na is serum sodium concentration (mmol/L)
  - **Note:** This formula estimates only the free water deficit, which is the volume of pure water required to normalize plasma sodium. It does not account for concomitant hypovolemia or other extracellular fluid deficits.[14]
- Current recommendations are to administer fluid to lower the serum sodium concentration by about 0.5–1.0 mEq/L per hour. Replace no more than half the free water deficit in the first 24 hours. Replace the remainder over the next 24–72 hours or more. Rapid replacement can cause cerebral edema.
- Normovolemic hypernatremia
  - Fluid replacement orally, via nasogastric tube, or IV (if necessary)
  - Evaluate for possible diabetes insipidus
- Hypovolemic hypernatremia (water deficit > sodium deficit)
  - Estimate the degree of volume depletion by using the water deficit formula.
  - If significant hypovolemia exists, use 0.9% normal saline to correct the intravascular volume deficit; 0.45% normal saline may then be used to correct the free water deficit.
  - If significant hypovolemia does not exist, use 0.45% normal saline to correct hypovolemia.
  - Recalculate the water deficit frequently during treatment, based on serial serum sodium measurements. Adjust the rate of fluid replacement therapy accordingly.
- Hypervolemic hypernatremia (sodium gains > water gains)
  - Remove the source of salt excess
  - Administer diuretics (e.g., furosemide) if inadequate spontaneous diuresis

---

[14] Reprinted from *Saunders Manual of Critical Care,* 1e, James A. Kruse, Mitchell P. Fink, & Richard W. Carlson, "Hypernatremia," Copyright 2003, with permission from Elsevier.

- Replace water
- Consider peritoneal dialysis or hemodialysis if renal function is markedly impaired.

Hyponatremia

Hyponatremic patients have an excess of free water as compared to sodium.

Causes

- The causes of hyponatremia can include any of the following:
  - Normovolemic hyponatremia
    - Psychogenic polydipsia
    - Administration of hypotonic IV or irrigation fluids in the immediate postoperative period
    - Infants given excessive amounts of free water
    - Renal failure
    - Hypothyroidism
    - Syndrome of inappropriate antidiuretic hormone secretion (SIADH)
  - Hypovolemic hyponatremia
    - GI losses (e.g., vomiting, diarrhea)
    - Excessive sweating
    - Addison's disease
    - Third spacing of fluids (e.g., peritonitis, pancreatitis, burns)
    - Use of thiazide diuretics, amiodarone, carbamazepine, opiates, oxytocin, selective serotonin reuptake inhibitors, or trazodone (among others)
    - Prolonged exercise in a hot environment with aggressive hydration of hypo-osmolar fluids (e.g., marathon runners, recreational hikers)
  - Hypervolemic hyponatremia
    - Acute or chronic renal failure
    - Hepatic cirrhosis
    - Congestive heart failure
    - Nephrotic syndrome
    - Consumption of large quantities of beer
    - MDMA (Ecstasy) use

Signs and Symptoms

The signs and symptoms of hyponatremia are related to the serum sodium concentration and how quickly the condition developed. Signs and symptoms are often absent until the serum sodium concentration is below 120 mEq/L.

- Mild-to-moderate hyponatremia
  - Usually asymptomatic
- Severe hyponatremia
  - Altered mental status and seizures

- Hypovolemic hyponatremia
  - Dry mucous membranes, tachycardia, poor skin turgor
  - Hypotension, shock
- Hypervolemic hyponatremia
  - Pulmonary crackles, S3 gallop
  - Peripheral edema, ascites

Treatment

- O_2, IV, monitor, vital signs
- Obtain serum osmolality, urine osmolality, and urine sodium to determine the cause of hyponatremia and help guide therapy.
- Determine if the patient is hypervolemic, hypovolemic, or normovolemic.
  - If normovolemic, restrict fluid intake to 1/2 to 1/3 maintenance fluid requirements and treat the underlying cause.
  - If hypovolemic, replace volume with 0.9% normal saline.
  - If hypervolemic, restrict water and initiate diuresis with furosemide.
  - In asymptomatic patients, the serum sodium concentration should be raised by no more than 0.5–1.0 mEq/L per hour and by less than 10–12 mEq/L over the first 24 hours. [15]
- Patients with severe hyponatremia and profound neurologic symptoms often require treatment with hypertonic (0.3%) saline solution.
  - Raise the serum sodium concentration at a rate of 1 mEq/L per hour for the first 3–4 hours or until seizures subside.[16]
  - Do not raise the serum sodium concentration more than 12 mEq/L during the first 24 hours.[17]
- Monitor fluid intake and output closely.
- Monitor the serum sodium level frequently to evaluate the progress of therapy and periodically recalculate fluid requirements.
- **Note:** Osmotic demyelination syndrome (ODS; also called central pontine myelinolysis) is a neurologic disorder associated with significant morbidity and mortality that typically begins 1–3 days after overly rapid correction of serum sodium.
  - ODS is characterized by dysarthria, dysphagia, seizures, altered mental status, flaccid paralysis, and hypotension. There is no specific treatment for ODS.
  - Patients at increased risk of ODS include alcoholics, elderly women taking thiazide diuretics, malnourished or hypokalemic patients, and burn patients.

---

[15] Adapted with permission from Gary G. Singer, Barry M. Brenner. Chapter 49: Fluid and Electrolyte Disturbances, in Harrison's Online (accessmedicine.com; *Harrison's Principles of Internal Medicine*, 15th ed.); Part 2: Cardinal Manifestations and Presentation of Diseases, Section 7: Alterations in Renal and Urinary Tract Function. Editors: Eugene Braunwald, Anthony S. Fauci, Kurt J. Isselbacher, et al. Copyright (c) 2001-2003 The McGraw-Hill Companies, Inc.
[16] Ibid.
[17] Ibid.

Calcium

Calcium is a critical element in many of the body's enzymatic reactions. It plays a role in nerve transmission, blood clotting, permeability of cell membranes, bone growth and formation, and muscle contraction. Approximately 99% of the body's calcium is found in the cells of the bones and teeth, and the remaining 1% is found in the extracellular fluid.

Almost half of extracellular calcium is ionized (or free) calcium—the physiologically active form of calcium in plasma. About 50% of the extracellular calcium is bound to plasma proteins, primarily albumin. The rest circulates bound to anions (e.g., phosphate, carbonate, citrate, lactate, and sulfate).[18]

In most cases, the hospital laboratory measures the total serum calcium level. This value reflects the total amount (protein-bound, complexed, ionized) of calcium in the blood. The normal value for total serum calcium is 8.5–10.5 mg/dL. Ionized calcium should be measured if a calcium excess or deficit is suspected. It is roughly 50% of the total serum calcium and ranges from 4.2 mg/dL to 4.8 mg/dL.

A significant amount of the extracellular calcium is bound to the plasma protein albumin, so the total serum calcium concentration is directly related to the albumin concentration. At a physiologic pH of 7.4, 1 g of albumin binds 0.8 mg/dL of calcium. A decrease in serum albumin of 1 g/dL leads to a total calcium decrease of 0.8 mg/dL. The normal serum albumin level is 4 g/dL. Because of this relationship, the total serum calcium concentration should be corrected when circulating albumin levels are abnormal to determine if treatment is warranted. Use the following formula to calculate a corrected (true) serum calcium level:[19]

$$\text{Measured calcium}_{total} + [(0.8) \times (\text{protein}_{normal} - \text{protein}_{measured})] = \text{corrected calcium}$$

For example, if a patient's total measured calcium is 8.8 mg/dL and his measured albumin level is 3 g/dL, his corrected calcium level is 9.6 mg/dL.

Using the formula:

$$8.8 \text{ mg/dL} + [(0.8) \times (4 - 3 \text{ g/dL})] = \text{corrected calcium}$$

$$9.6 \text{ mg/dL} = \text{corrected calcium}$$

the corrected calcium value is in the normal range (8.5–10.5 mg/dL), and the patient would most likely not be treated.

Serum pH also influences serum calcium levels. Acidosis (a decrease in serum pH) decreases calcium binding to albumin and results in increased ionized calcium. Alkalosis (an increase in serum pH) increases calcium binding to albumin and results in decreased ionized calcium.

Hypercalcemia

Hypercalcemic ECG changes are illustrated in Figure 10-8.

---

[18] K. L. McCance and S. E. Heuther, *Pathophysiology: The Biologic Basis for Disease in Adults and Children,* 4th ed. (Mosby, 2002).

[19] Reprinted from Rosen's Emergency Medicine: Concepts and Clinical Practice, 5e, M.A. Gibbs, A.B. Wolfson, & V.S. Tayal, "Electrolyte Disturbances," Copyright 2002, with permission from Elsevier.

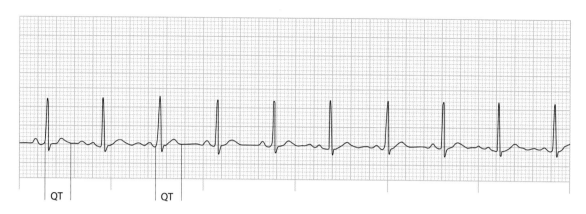

FIGURE 10-8 Hypercalcemia.

Causes

- The causes of hypercalcemia can include any of the following:
  - Endocrine disorders
    - Hyperparathyroidism
    - Hyperthyroidism
    - Adrenal insufficiency
    - Pheochromocytoma
  - Cancer or tumors
  - Medications (e.g., lithium, thiazide diuretics, theophylline, estrogens for breast cancer)
  - Tuberculosis
  - Vitamin D or vitamin A toxicity
  - Paget's disease of bone, immobilization
  - Milk-alkali syndrome
  - Renal failure

Signs and Symptoms

- Mild elevations in calcium levels
  - Few or no symptoms
- Total calcium levels of 12 to < 15 mg/dL
  - Weakness, fatigue, emotional lability, and confusion
- Total calcium levels of 15 to < 20 mg/dL
  - Weakness, disorientation, confusion, lethargy, and coma
- ECG changes associated with hypercalcemia may include a shortened QT interval, prolonged PR and QRS intervals, an increased QRS voltage, and T-wave flattening and widening.

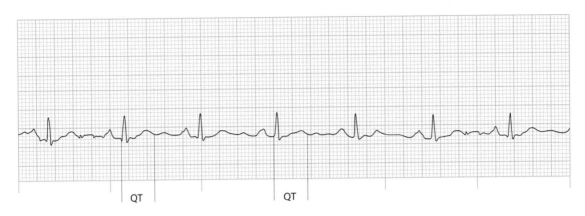

QT   QT

FIGURE 10-9   Hypocalcemia.

Treatment
- O$_2$, IV, monitor, vital signs
- Moderate hypercalcemia (12 to $<$ 15 mg/dL), with symptoms
- Severe hypercalcemia (total calcium concentration $\geq$ 15 mg/dL) :
  - Hydrate the patient.
    - Restores volume, decreases the calcium level through dilution, and increases renal calcium clearance (if there is adequate renal function)
    - Infuse 0.9% normal saline at 300–500 mL/hr until fluid deficits are corrected (urine output $\geq$ 200 mL/hr), and then decrease the infusion rate to 100–200 mL/hr.
  - Consider hemodialysis.
    - Rapidly decreases calcium levels
  - Inhibit calcium release from bones.
    - Drugs such as calcitonin, pamidronate (Aredia), and etidronate (Didronel) inhibit the action of osteoclasts in bone, reducing bone reabsorption of calcium.
  - Treat the underlying illness.
  - Induce diuresis with furosemide.
    - Controversial
    - May increase the release of calcium from the bones

Hypocalcemia
The relationship between calcium, potassium, and magnesium is critical to maintain adequate serum calcium levels. Hypocalcemic ECG changes are illustrated in Figure 10-9.

Causes
- The causes of hypocalcemia can include any of the following:
  - Hypoparathyroidism

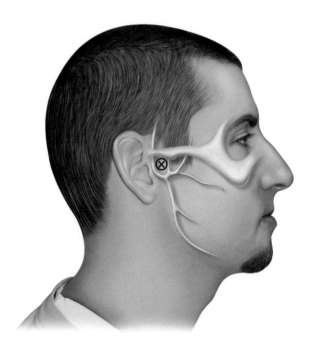

FIGURE 10-10   Chvostek's sign. Chvostek's sign is elicited by tapping along the course of the facial nerve (just anterior to the ear, below the zygomatic bone). A positive response is evidenced by twitching of the facial muscles on that side.

- Vitamin D deficiency
- Renal tubular disease
- Other electrolyte disturbances
  - Magnesium depletion
  - Hyperphosphatemia
- Acute pancreatitis
- Hypoproteinemia
- Sepsis, toxic shock syndrome
- Medications (e.g., cimetidine, glucagon, norepinephrine, loop diuretics, nitroprusside, phenytoin, phenobarbital, heparin)

Signs and Symptoms
- Mild hypocalcemia
  - Frequently asymptomatic
- Ionized calcium less than 2.5 mg/dL
  - Neuromuscular irritability
    - Muscle cramps in the back and legs
    - Paresthesias of the face, fingers, or toes
    - Positive Chvostek's sign (Figure 10-10)
    - Positive Trousseau's sign (Figure 10-11)

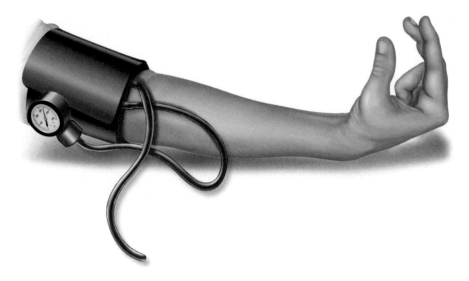

FIGURE 10-11   Trousseau's sign. Trousseau's sign is present when carpal spasm results when a BP cuff remains inflated for minutes to a pressure 20 mm Hg above the patient's systolic blood pressure. A positive Trousseau's sign may also be seen in alkalosis, hypomagnesemia, hypokalemia, hyperkalemia, and rarely, when there is no electrolyte disturbance.

- Severe hypocalcemia
  - May cause tetany, laryngospasm, or generalized convulsions
  - Decreased myocardial contractility
  - Heart failure
- ECG changes
  - Prolongation of the QT interval
  - T-wave inversion
  - VT, TdP
  - Bradycardia and AV blocks

Treatment

- O_2, IV, monitor, vital signs
- Acute hypocalcemia is treated with calcium gluconate or calcium chloride. Administer calcium slowly by IV. Rapid administration may result in syncope, hypotension, and cardiac arrhythmias, including severe bradycardia.
  - Calcium gluconate
    - Less irritating to tissues than calcium chloride
    - For symptomatic hypocalcemia, give 93–186 mg (10–20 mL) of 10% solution IV over 10 minutes.
    - Follow with an IV infusion of 540–720 mg (58–77 mL) of 10% calcium gluconate in 500–1000 mL D5W. Infuse at a rate of 0.5–2.0 mg/kg/hr.

- Calcium chloride
    - Contains three times as much available calcium as calcium gluconate
    - Can cause severe thrombophlebitis and tissue burns if extravasated
    - For symptomatic hypocalcemia, give 5 mL of 10% solution IV over 10 minutes.
    - If indicated, administer 10 mL of 10% calcium chloride by IV infusion in the next 6–12 hours.
    - Infusion over long time periods is not recommended.
- Observe closely for cardiac arrhythmias, particularly in patients taking digitalis.
- Measure the serum calcium every 4–6 hours. The goal is to maintain total serum calcium concentration between 7 and 9 mg/dL.
- Correct magnesium, potassium, and pH abnormalities.
- In hypocalcemic cardiac arrest:
    - Administer normal saline IV bolus
    - Administer calcium gluconate *or* calcium chloride IV
        - Calcium gluconate: Give 279 mg (30 mL) of 10% solution IVP over 1–3 minutes.
        - Calcium chloride: Give 10 mL of 10% solution IVP over 1–3 minutes.[20]

Magnesium

Magnesium is the fourth most abundant cation in the body. Almost half of the body's magnesium is stored in the muscles and bones. Extracellular fluid contains about 1% of total body magnesium, and the rest is found in the intracellular fluid. One-half of extracellular magnesium is ionized, and approximately 30% is bound to serum albumin. The normal plasma magnesium concentration ranges from 1.35 mEq/L to 2.20 mEq/L. Because < 1% of the body's magnesium is present in the extracellular fluid, serum levels do not necessarily reflect the status of total body stores of magnesium.

Hypermagnesemia

Causes

- The causes of hypermagnesemia can include any of the following:
    - Renal failure
    - Bowel obstruction
    - Excess magnesium administration
    - Untreated ketoacidosis

Signs and Symptoms

- Serum magnesium level 3 to < 4 mEq/L
    - Nausea/vomiting

---

[20] Ibid.

- Flushing
- Lethargy, weakness, dizziness
- Mild hypotension
- Serum magnesium level 4 to < 5 mEq/L
  - Diminished deep tendon reflexes
  - Increasing muscle weakness
- Serum magnesium level 5 to < 8 mEq/L
  - Somnolence
  - ECG changes
  - Worsening hypotension
  - Loss of deep tendon reflexes
- Serum magnesium level ≥ 8 mEq/L
  - Complete AV block
  - Coma
  - Respiratory arrest, cardiac arrest
- ECG signs
  - Increased PR and QT intervals
  - Decreased P wave voltage, tall T waves, and increased QRS duration
  - Cardiac arrhythmias may include complete AV block and asystole

Treatment

- O$_2$, IV, monitor, vital signs
- Treatment depends on the underlying cause, the severity of hypermagnesemia, and the patient's clinical presentation.
  - Discontinue any sources of magnesium.
  - Administer IV fluids to dilute the serum magnesium concentration and increase urine output.
  - Administer calcium gluconate or calcium chloride to treat the signs and symptoms caused by excess magnesium levels.
    - Administer *either* calcium gluconate 10 mL of a 10% solution *or* calcium chloride 5–10 mL of a 10% solution IV over 5–10 minutes.[21]
  - Remove excess magnesium from the body.
    - If renal function is normal, consider the use of a loop diuretic (e.g., furosemide) and IV infusions of normal saline to induce diuresis and promote magnesium excretion.
- Carefully monitor the patient's magnesium level and ECG.
- Dialysis is indicated for severe hypermagnesemia.

---

[21] Ibid.

Hypomagnesemia

Causes

- The causes of hypomagnesemia can include any of the following:
  - Alcoholism
  - Malnutrition or malabsorption syndromes
  - Burns
  - GI losses (e.g., pancreatitis, diarrhea, bowel resection)
  - Renal disease
  - Hypothermia
  - Diabetic ketoacidosis
  - Medications (e.g., loop and thiazide diuretics, gentamicin, digoxin)
  - Hypercalcemia, and phosphate deficiency
  - Hyperthyroidism, hypothyroidism

Signs and Symptoms

- Tremors, twitching, tetany, and hyperactive deep tendon reflexes, nystagmus
- Ataxia, seizures
- Altered mental status, depression, confusion, seizures, emotional lability, and hallucinations
- Positive Chvostek's and Trousseau's signs may be present
- ECG signs
  - Prolonged PR and QT intervals
  - ST-segment depression
  - Prolonged QRS duration
  - T-wave inversion
  - PVCs, SVT, VT, VF, and TdP

Treatment

- O$_2$, IV, monitor, vital signs
- Treatment depends on the underlying cause, the severity of hypomagnesemia, and the patient's clinical presentation.
  - Mild or chronic hypomagnesemia
    - Oral replacement therapy. If symptoms are severe, IV magnesium administration is indicated.
  - Severe symptomatic hypomagnesemia
    - Give 1–2 g magnesium sulfate IV over 5–20 minutes.[22]

---

[22] American Heart Association, "AHA Guidelines for Cardiopulmonary Resuscitation and Emergency Cardiovascular Care," *Circulation* 112, suppl. 1 (2005).

- Carefully monitor the patient's magnesium level, ECG, respiratory status, and deep tendon reflexes. Patients with renal failure should be monitored carefully to prevent hypermagnesemia.
- Magnesium is available in various concentrations. For safety, be sure the physician's order clearly indicates the concentration to be used.
- Measure serum calcium. Hypocalcemia often accompanies hypomagnesemia.

The Bottom Line

The management of patients with complicated medical and traumatic disorders can be very complex. You must have a basic understanding of these conditions and use appropriate reference materials to guide your care.

Appendices

ACLS Medications Table

This appendix lists selected information about drugs used in the care of a patient with an Advanced Cardiac Life Support emergency. Before using these drugs, the healthcare provider is expected to be familiar with all contraindications, drug interactions, and pregnancy risks associated with the use of the drug. Side effects listed are those that occur most frequently.

Medications and medication details for the experienced provider are provided in italics.

Drug	Action, Uses, Adult Dose, Side Effects (SE), Notes
Acetylsalicylic acid (aspirin)	**Action:** Prostaglandin inhibitor; inhibits platelet aggregation **Uses:** Should be given as soon as possible to all patients suspected of having an ACS unless contraindications present **Adult dose:** 162–325 mg PO (chewed if possible); may give 300 mg rectal suppository **SE:** Bleeding, stomach pain, heartburn, nausea, vomiting, allergy **Notes:** Ask patient to chew to hasten absorption.
Activated charcoal (Liqui-Char)	***Action:*** *Antidote; physically binds (adsorbs) toxins from GI tract* ***Uses:*** *Oral ingestion of toxic substances* ***Adult dose:*** *1–2 g/kg by mouth or via gastric tube, up to 50–100 g* ***SE:*** *May induce vomiting in some patients; may worsen overdose-induced ileus; may cause constipation and mechanical bowel obstruction when used in multiple doses* ***Notes:*** *Most useful if administered within 1 hour of ingestion. In cases of sustained-released agents, repeated doses (0.5 g/kg every 4 hours) may be beneficial. Charcoal stains clothing, walls, floors, ceilings, etc. Contraindicated in ingestion of caustics. Relatively contraindicated in cases of hydrocarbon ingestion. Ineffective for ingestion of iron, lithium, heavy metals, and other ions.*

Adenosine (Adenocard)	**Action:** Antiarrhythmic; slows AV node conduction; interrupts AV nodal reentry pathways
	Uses: Most forms of PSVT
	Adult dose: 6 mg initially. If arrhythmia is not corrected, give 12 mg; may repeat another 12-mg dose once. Give each dose as rapid IVP over 1–3 sec. Follow with 20 mL NS flush. Wait 1–2 min. between doses.
	SE: Facial flushing, lightheadedness, paresthesias, headache, diaphoresis, palpitations, chest pain, hypotension, nausea, shortness of breath, bronchospasm
	Notes: Half-life < 10 sec; theophylline and methylxanthines reduce effect; dipyridamole potentiates effect; transient arrhythmias common after termination of PSVT; does not convert atrial fibrillation/flutter or ventricular tachycardia, do not use in WPW.
Albuterol (Proventil, Ventolin)	***Action:*** *Moderately selective beta-2 receptor agonist*
	Uses: *Acute bronchospasm, asthma, bronchospasm prophylaxis, hyperkalemia*
	Adult dose:
	• *Acute bronchospasm/asthma: 2.5 mg every 6–8 hours as needed over 5–15 min. For severe episodes, 2.5–5.0 mg initially every 20 min. for 3 doses, then 2.5–10.0 mg every 1–4 hours as needed, or 10–15 mg/hr by continuous nebulization.*
	• *Hyperkalemia: 10–20 mg nebulized over 15 min.; may repeat (unlabeled use)*
	SE: *Anxiety, arrhythmia exacerbation, excitability, hypokalemia, irritability, palpitations, restlessness, ST-T wave changes, throat irritation, tremor*
	Notes: *Nebulized albuterol lowers the serum potassium level for at least 2 hours; takes 10–20 min. to work and has high side effect incidence.*
Alteplase (tPA)	**Action:** Fibrinolytic; converts plasminogen to plasmin, promoting fibrinolysis
	Uses: ST-segment-elevation MI, acute ischemic stroke
	Adult dose (MI dose):
	• 100 mg total dose. Initial bolus 15-mg IVP over 1–2 min. Follow with 0.75 mg/kg (maximum 50 mg) infused over next 30 min., and then 0.5 mg/kg (maximum 35 mg) infused over the next 60 min.
	• (Stroke dose): 0.9 mg/kg (maximum 90 mg) total dose over 60 min. Give 10% of total dose IVP over 1 min., and then 90% of the total dose over 60 min.
	SE: Bleeding, arrhythmias, bruising (especially at venipuncture sites)
	Notes: Must meet specific inclusion/exclusion criteria for STEMI or stroke. Stop drug administration if bleeding occurs.

(continued)

Amiodarone (Cordarone)	**Action:** Class III antiarrhythmic; blocks sodium, potassium, and calcium channels; blocks alpha- and beta-adrenergic receptors; prolongs action potential in all cardiac tissues, including bypass tracts
	Uses: VF/pulseless VT unresponsive to CPR, shock, or pressors; atrial fibrillation/flutter; stable narrow-complex tachycardias; stable VT; nausea; cardiogenic shock
	Adult dose:
	• Cardiac arrest: 300 mg IVP/IO; dilute in 20–30 mL D5W. May repeat in 3–5 min. with 150 mg IVP/IO once.
	• Other indications: Rapid IV infusion of 150 mg over 10 min. followed by an IV infusion of 1 mg/min for 6 hours, then 0.5 mg/min for 18 hours. If needed, the rapid IV infusion of 150 mg may be repeated every 10 min.
	SE: Hypotension, bradycardia, AV block, may prolong QT interval
	Notes: Seek expert consultation for uses other than ventricular fibrillation or ventricular tachycardia. Extremely long half-life; maximum cumulative dose is 2.2 g IV/24 hours.
Angiotensin-converting enzyme (ACE) inhibitors **Captopril (Capoten), Enalapril (Vasotec), Lisinopril (Prinivil, Zestril), Ramipril (Altace), and Others**	**Action:** Antihypertensives; lower blood pressure by interrupting the renin-angiotensin-aldosterone cycle; decrease preload and afterload
	Uses: Suspected MI especially if hypertension, heart failure without hypotension, and/or ejection fraction less than 40% is present
	Adult dose:
	• Captopril (oral): Initial dose 6.25 mg; increase to 25 mg TID. Target dose 50 mg TID as tolerated.
	• Enalapril
	• Oral: Start with a single dose of 2.5 mg. Increase slowly as tolerated to a maximum of 20 mg BID.
	• IV (Enalaprilat): 1.25 mg IV every 6 hours. Give slowly IV over at least 5 min.
	• Lisinopril (oral): First dose 5 mg within 24 hours of symptom onset. Then 5 mg after 24 hours, 10 mg after 48 hours, and then 10 mg daily.
	• Ramipril (oral): Begin with single dose of 2.5 mg. Titrate to 5 mg BID as tolerated.
	SE: Anaphylactoid reactions, syncope, chest discomfort, fatigue, dyspepsia, headache, hypotension, cough, dizziness
	Notes: Adjust dose in patients with renal impairment or renal failure. IV administration of ACE inhibitors is contraindicated within the first 24 hours after an MI.

Atenolol (Tenormin)	**Action:** Cardio-selective beta-blocker **Uses:** STEMI, NSTEMI, unstable angina **Adult dose:** 5 mg IV over 5 min. May give second dose after 10 min. **SE:** Bradycardia, dizziness, fatigue, nausea, dyspnea, hypotension **Notes:** Concurrent use with calcium channel blockers can cause severe hypotension. Do not use if the patient is bradycardic.
Atropine sulfate	**Action:** Parasympathetic blocker; suppresses vagus-mediated bradycardia, blocks acetylcholine at parasympathetic sites. **Uses:** Symptomatic sinus bradycardia, AV block at the level of the AV node, asystole, PEA (if rate is slow), *organophosphate or carbamate poisoning* **Adult dose:** • Asystole/PEA: 1 mg IVP, may repeat every 3–5 min., up to 3 doses to a maximum dose of 3 mg. ET dose: 2–3 mg • Bradycardia: 0.5 mg IVP; may repeat every 3–5 min., to a total dose of 3 mg. • *Organophosphate/carbamate poisoning: Starting dose is 2–4 mg IVP every 5 min.; endpoint is drying of secretions or signs of toxicity.* **SE:** Anticholinergic effects, tachycardia, delirium with excessive doses, paradoxical bradycardia if administered in doses of < 0.5 mg **Notes:** Increases myocardial oxygen demand. Use with caution in the presence of myocardial ischemia and hypoxia. *Atropine does not reverse muscle paralysis and fasciculations seen with organophosphate insecticides.*
Calcium chloride	**Action:** *Electrolyte* **Uses:** *ECG changes related to known or suspected hyperkalemia, calcium channel blocker overdose, or prophylaxis before IV administration of calcium channel blocker* **Adult dose:** • *Hyperkalemia and hypermagnesemia: 500–1000 mg (5–10 mL of a 10% solution) IV over 2–5 min.* • *Hypocalcemia: 500 mg (5 mL of a 10% solution) IV over 10 min.; follow with 36.6 mL of a 10% solution IV over 6–12 hours (monitor calcium levels).* • *Calcium channel blocker overdose 500–1000 mg (5–10 mL of a 10% solution) IV over 10 min. Repeat as needed.* **SE:** *Rapid injection may cause the patient to complain of a tingling sensation or "heat waves"; peripheral vasodilation* **Notes:** *Do not mix with sodium bicarbonate. Avoid use if digoxin toxicity is suspected.*

(continued)

Cimetidine (Tagamet)	**Action:** *Histamine-2 blocker; reversible histamine antagonist at parietal cells, inhibits gastric acid secretion* **Uses:** *Anaphylaxis (unlabeled use), gastroesophageal reflux disease (GERD), duodenal or gastric ulcer, Zollinger-Ellison Syndrome* **Adult dose:** *300 mg PO, IM, or IV (dilute with 18 mL NS and administer over 5 min. IV) every 6–8 hours; not to exceed 2400 mg/day.* **SE:** *Diarrhea, hepatitis, dizziness, sleepiness, headache, confusion, delirium, hallucinations, double vision, ataxia, hypotension and arrhythmias following rapid IV administration* **Notes:** *Confusion is more likely to occur in geriatric patients with impaired renal or hepatic function.*
Clopidogrel (Plavix)	**Action:** Antiplatelet agent; inhibits platelet aggregation through irreversible modification of the platelet ADP receptor **Uses:** Non-ST-segment-elevation MI (NSTEMI), unstable angina **Adult dose:** 300 mg PO, then 75 mg PO daily for patients with ST-segment depression or dynamic T-wave inversion **SE:** Severe rash, upper respiratory infection, chest pain, headache, dizziness, arthralgia, bleeding, cough, pruritis **Notes:** Consider for patients with NSTEMI and unstable angina if in-hospital conservative approach is planned *or* cardiac catheterization and PCI are planned and the risk for bleeding is not high.
Diazepam (Valium)	**Action:** Benzodiazepine, sedative, anticonvulsant **Uses:** Transient sedation/amnesia for medical procedures (e.g., cardioversion, pacing); cocaine-induced supraventricular arrhythmias (PSVT, rapid atrial fibrillation and atrial flutter), cocaine-induced ventricular tachycardia, cocaine-induced hypertension, cocaine-induced ACS; seizures; status epilepticus **Adult dose:** Premedication before cardioversion: 5–15 mg slow IV. Administer no faster than 2 mg/min. *Seizures: 5–10 mg IV over 2 min. every 10–20 min. to a maximum of 30 mg in 8 hours.* *Cocaine toxicity: 5 mg slow IV, repeat as needed to 20 mg* **SE:** Bradycardia, hypotension, phlebitis, vascular spasm, respiratory depression, ataxia **Notes:** Do not administer faster than 5 mg/min IV in adults to avoid respiratory arrest. Avoid small veins such as those on the dorsum of the hand or wrist; reduce the dose in the elderly.

Digoxin Immune FAB (Digibind)	***Action:*** *Antidote, antigen-binding fragments bind and inactivate digoxin or digitoxin* ***Uses:*** *Digoxin toxicity associated with the following: severe ventricular dysrhythmias, hemodynamically significant bradydysrhythmias unresponsive to atropine, serum potassium > 5 mEq/L with signs or symptoms of digoxin toxicity[1]* ***Adult dose:*** *Formulas for calculating the dose are available in the package insert. In acute poisoning, 5–15 vials are usually required (average dose 10 vials; up to 20 vials may be required). For toxicity related to chronic ingestion, 3–5 vials is usually adequate.* ***SE:*** *Anaphylaxis, erythema, urticaria, and facial edema; hypokalemia; exacerbation of CHF; increase in ventricular rate with atrial fibrillation. Do not use in patients with allergy to sheep.* ***Notes:*** *Administer calculated dose IV over 30 min.*
Digoxin (Lanoxin, Lanoxicaps)	**Action:** Cardiac glycoside; increases myocardial contractility; depresses impulse conduction through SA and AV nodes **Uses:** To slow ventricular response rate in stable patients with atrial fibrillation or atrial flutter **Adult dose:** Loading dose of 10–15 mcg/kg lean body weight IV over 5 min.; maintenance dose affected by body size and renal function. **SE:** Visual disturbances, fatigue, weakness, nausea, loss of appetite, abdominal discomfort, dizziness, headache, diarrhea, vomiting, arrhythmias **Notes:** Limited use in emergency cardiac care. Reduce dose by 50% if concurrent amiodarone use. Possible toxicity if used concurrently with many drugs. Do not repeat dose for 4–6 hours. Do not use if the patient has AV block or idiopathic constrictive pericarditis. Therapeutic serum level 0.8–2.0 ng/mL.
Diltiazem (Cardizem)	**Action:** Calcium channel blocker; inhibits the movement of calcium ions across cell membranes, decreasing myocardial contractility. **Uses:** PSVT, atrial fibrillation/flutter with rapid ventricular rate **Adult dose:** 15–20 mg (0.25 mg/kg) IV over 2 min. May repeat in 15 min. with 20–25 mg (0.35 mg/kg) IV over 2 min. Maintenance infusion 5–15 mg/hr titrated to heart rate. **SE:** Hypotension, bradycardia, arrhythmia, injection-site reactions (e.g., itching, burning), flushing **Notes:** Avoid in wide-complex tachycardia caused by toxicity, of unknown type, or in patients with WPW. Do not use in patients with sick sinus syndrome, AV block, hypotension, or pulmonary congestion.

(continued)

---

[1]"Common Cardiovascular Drugs," in *Rosen's Emergency Medicine: Concepts and Clinical Practice,* 5th ed., ed.-in-chief John A. Marx, chap. 146 (Mosby, 2002).

Diphenhydramine (Benadryl)	**Action:** *Antihistamine* **Uses:** *Anaphylaxis, phenothiazine reactions* **Adult dose:** *10–50 mg IV (each 25 mg or less over at least 1 min.) or deep IM* **SE:** *Thickening of bronchial secretions, chest tightness, wheezing; nasal stuffiness, sedation; in elderly hypotension* **Notes:** *Onset of action IV is 5–10 min. Do not use in an acute asthma attack.*
Dobutamine (Dobutrex)	**Action:** Positive inotrope; increases myocardial contractility **Uses:** Acute pulmonary edema with systolic blood pressure of 70–100 mm Hg and *no* signs of shock **Adult dose:** 2–20 mcg/kg/min IV infusion **SE:** Tachycardia, ventricular ectopy, excessive increase in BP **Notes:** Titrate so heart rate does not increase by > 10% of baseline; do not mix with sodium bicarbonate. Do not use in patients with idiopathic hypertrophic subaortic stenosis or if sensitivity to sulfites.
Dopamine (Intropin)	**Action:** Sympathomimetic; stimulates alpha and beta receptors of the heart **Uses:** Symptomatic bradycardia, hypotension (systolic BP 70–100 mm Hg) not due to hypovolemia **Adult dose:** 2–20 mcg/kg/min IV infusion **SE:** Arrhythmias, hypertension, hypotension at low doses, nausea/vomiting, headache, dyspnea, tachycardia, vasoconstriction **Notes:** Onset of action is 2–5 min. Do not use in patients with sulfites sensitivity, pheochromocytoma, or during ventricular fibrillation.
Epinephrine (Adrenalin)	**Action:** Sympathomimetic; alpha receptor stimulation increases coronary and cerebral perfusion pressure **Uses:** Cardiac arrest, symptomatic bradycardia, *anaphylaxis, severe asthma* **Adult dose:** • Cardiac arrest: 1 mg (1:10,000) IVP every 3–5 min.; ET dose 2.0–2.5 mg (dilute in 10 mL NS). • *Cardiac arrest if beta-blocker or calcium channel toxicity present: Up to 0.2 mg/kg IVP* • Bradycardia: 2–10 mcg/min. IV infusion • *Anaphylaxis: 0.3–0.5 mg (1:1000) IM; may repeat in 15–20 min. if no clinical improvement* • *Anaphylaxis with immediate life threat: 0.1 mg (1:10,000) slow IV over 5 min.* • *Severe acute asthma: Usual dose 0.3 mg (1:1000) SC; may repeat every 20 min. up to three times (total maximum dose 0.01 mg/kg).*

Epinephrine (Adrenalin) *(continued)*	**SE:** Increases myocardial oxygen demand, palpitations, tachycardia, tremors, anxiety, angina, headache **Notes:** Onset: IM 3–5 min., SC 5–10 min., IV immediate. Increase time interval between doses in arrest related to sympathomimetic poisoning.
Esmolol (Brevibloc)	**Action:** Class II antiarrhythmic agent; beta-blocker **Uses:** ST-segment-elevation MI, non-ST-segment-elevation MI, unstable angina **Adult dose:** • Loading infusion of 500 mcg/kg/min (0.5 mg/kg/min) IV over 1 min. followed by a 4-minute IV maintenance infusion of 50 mcg/kg/min (0.05 mg/kg/min). Maximum 200 mcg/kg/min (0.2 mg/kg/min). • If initial dosing inadequate, repeat IV loading dose of 500 mcg/kg/min (0.5 mg/kg/min) over 1 min. followed by infusion of 100 mcg/kg/min (0.1 mg/kg/min); maximum infusion rate of 300 mcg/kg/min (0.3 mg/kg/min) **SE:** Hypotension, bradycardia, dizziness, fatigue, nausea, dyspnea, sweating, pain at injection site **Notes:** Concurrent use with calcium channel blockers can cause severe hypotension.
Etomidate (Amidate)	**Action:** *Sedative/hypnotic* **Uses:** *Induction agent for rapid sequence intubation* **Adult dose:** *0.2–0.6 mg/kg IV over 30–60 sec.* **SE:** *Anaphylactoid reactions, apnea, hiccups, hypertension, hypotension, injection site reaction, laryngospasm, nausea/vomiting, respiratory depression, sinus bradycardia, sinus tachycardia, tachypnea, transient muscle movements* **Notes:** *Ultrashort acting*
Furosemide (Lasix)	**Action:** Loop diuretic; inhibits sodium and water absorption in the ascending loop of Henle and proximal and distal tubules **Uses:** Acute pulmonary edema, hypertensive emergencies, ascites, *hyperkalemia (unlabeled use)* **Adult dose:** • Pulmonary edema, hypertensive emergencies: 0.5–1.0 mg/kg IV over 1–2 min.; maximum 2 mg/kg • *Hyperkalemia: 40–80 mg IV over 1–2 min.* **SE:** Dehydration, hypokalemia, hypotension, hypovolemia, nausea, dyspepsia **Notes:** Give no faster than 20 mg/min.

(continued)

Glucagon	**Action:** *Reverses myocardial depression; enhances myocardial contractility, heart rate, and AV conduction; helps counteract hypoglycemia induced by beta-blocker overdose* **Uses:** *Beta-blocker toxicity; calcium channel blocker toxicity; anaphylaxis (all unlabeled uses)* **Adult dose:** • *Beta-blocker or calcium channel blocker overdose: 3 mg IV over 3 min. If the response to the IV bolus is favorable, begin an infusion of 3 mg/hr.* • *Anaphylaxis: 1–2 mg IM or slow IVP every 5 min. or 1–5 mg/hr* **SE:** *Nausea/vomiting (may increase vagal tone), mild hyperglycemia, hypokalemia, allergic reactions* **Notes:** *Short half-life (20 min.). Use D5W (not saline) to dilute when large doses of glucagon are administered because the standard 0.2% phenol diluent may worsen myocardial depression. Do not use if patient has pheochromocytoma.*
Glycoprotein IIb/IIIa Inhibitors (abciximab [ReoPro], eptifibatide [Integrilin], tirofiban [Aggrastat])	**Action:** Antiplatelet; interferes with platelet aggregation through glycoprotein IIb/IIIa inhibition **Uses:** Acute coronary syndromes (ACS) without ST-segment elevation **Adult dose:** • Abciximab: NSTEMI or unstable angina with planned PCI within 24 hours—0.25 mg/kg IVP (10–60 min. before procedure) followed by 0.125 mcg/kg/min IV infusion (maximum 10 mcg/min); During PCI—0.25 mg/kg IVP followed by infusion of 10 mcg/min. • Eptifibatide: ACS - 180 mcg/kg IV over 1–2 min. then 2 mcg/kg/min IV infusion; During PCI - 180 mcg/kg IV over 1–2 min. followed by IV infusion of 2 mcg/kg/min; repeat bolus in 10 min. • Tirofiban: ACS or PCI—0.4 mcg/kg/min IV infusion for 30 min., then 0.1 mcg/kg/min IV infusion **SE:** Increased bleeding tendencies, hypotension, palpitations, nausea **Notes:** Stop drug administration if bleeding or hypersensitivity occurs.
Heparin sodium, unfractionated (Liquaemin Sodium)	**Action:** Anticoagulant; reacts with antithrombin III to inactivate thrombin and inhibit thromboplastin formation **Uses:** Acute MI; use with fibrinolytics **Adult dose:** • STEMI: 60 IU/kg IV over 1 min. (maximum bolus 4000 IU) followed by 12 IU/kg/hr IV infusion (maximum 1000 IU/hr for patients > 70 kg). Adjust if needed to maintain activated partial thromboplastin time (aPTT) at 1.5–2.0 times control (50–70 sec) for 48 hours or until angiography.

- NSTEMI: 60–70 IU/kg IV over 1 min. (maximum bolus 5000 IU) followed by 12–15 IU/kg/hr infusion (maximum 1000 IU/hr)

SE: Bleeding, itching, transient thrombocytopenia

Notes: Check aPTT at 6, 12, 18, and 24 hours; monitor to ensure platelet count is never < 100,000. Increased risk of bleeding if other anticoagulants, aspirin, antiplatelets, or cephalosporins used concurrently. Do not use if there is uncontrolled bleeding.

Heparin–Low molecular weight (Bivalirudin [Angiomax], Dalteparin [Fragmin], Enoxaparin [Lovenox])	**Action:** Anticoagulant; reacts with antithrombin III to inactivate thrombin and inhibit thromboplastin formation **Uses:** Unstable angina, non-ST segment-elevation MI (NSTEMI) **Adult dose:** • Enoxaparin NSTEMI: 1 mg/kg every 12 hours SC. A bolus dose of 30 mg IV may be given prior to the first dose. • Enoxaparin STEMI (with fibrinolytic therapy): 30 mg IV followed by 1 mg/kg SC twice daily until discharged. • Bivalirudin: During PCI - 0.25 mg/kg IV followed by 0.5 mg/kg/hr for 12 hours, then 0.25 mg/kg/hr for 36 hours. Infusion rate should be decreased if aPTT > 75 seconds during first 12 hours. **SE:** Bleeding, itching, rash, thrombocytopenia, back pain, nausea, headache **Notes:** Oral aspirin therapy should be given concurrently. Contraindicated in patients with hypersensitivity to heparin or pork products and in patients with active major bleeding. May not be appropriate for patients older than 75 years or with renal insufficiency. Monitor aPTT and adjust dose if needed.
Ibutilide (Corvert)	**Action:** Class III antiarrhythmic **Uses:** For rapid conversion of atrial fibrillation or atrial flutter to sinus rhythm (if onset < 48 hours) **Adult dose:** • Patients weighing ≥ 60 kg: 1 mg IV infused over 10 min. • Patients weighing < 60 kg: 0.01 mg/kg IV infused over 10 min. • If the arrhythmia does not terminate within 10 min. after the end of the initial infusion (regardless of body weight), a second 10-minute infusion of equal strength may be given 10 min. after completion of the first infusion. **SE:** Monomorphic or polymorphic VT, hypotension, bundle branch block, AV block, bradycardia, QT interval prolongation, headache **Notes:** May cause potentially fatal arrhythmias, especially sustained polymorphic VT. Do not administer to patients with prolonged QT interval.

(continued)

Inamrinone (Inocor)	**Action:** *Cardiac inotropic agent; phosphodiesterase III inhibitor with vasodilator activity* **Uses:** *Severe CHF unresponsive to digitalis, diuretics, and/or vasodilators* **Adult dose:** *0.75 mg/kg IV loading dose slowly over 10–15 min. Based on the clinical response, an additional loading dose of 0.75 mg/kg may be given 30 min. after initiation of therapy. Follow with IV infusion of 5–15 mcg/kg/min, titrated to effect.* **SE:** *Tachyarrhythmias, hypotension, thrombocytopenia, nausea* **Notes:** *Do not mix with dextrose solutions or other drugs; do not exceed a daily dose of 10 mg/kg. Do not use in patients with bisulfite sensitivity.*
Ipratropium bromide (Atrovent)	**Action:** *Anticholinergic; blocks acetylcholine effects on bronchioles and causes bronchodilation* **Uses:** *Bronchospasm in COPD/asthma* **Adult dose:** *0.5 mg in 2.5 mL normal saline by small-volume nebulizer* **SE:** *Headache, cough, nausea, dry mouth* **Notes:** *Can be used either alone or in combination with other bronchodilators, especially beta-adrenergics (e.g., albuterol).*
Isoproterenol (Isuprel)	**Action:** Sympathomimetic; beta-1 and beta-2 stimulant effects **Uses:** • Temporizing measure before pacing for torsades de pointes unresponsive to other agents • Symptomatic bradycardia when atropine and dopamine or epinephrine have failed and pacing is not available • Temporary bradycardia management in heart transplant patients (denervated heart unresponsive to atropine) • Beta-adrenergic blocker poisoning **Adult dose:** 2–10 mcg/min IV infusion titrated to effect **SE:** Arrhythmias, hypotension, precipitation of angina pectoris, facial flushing, nervousness **Notes:** Onset: 1–5 min.; increases myocardial oxygen demand; do not give with epinephrine – can cause VF/VT; do not use for drug toxicity (except beta-blocker)
Ketamine (Ketalar)	**Action:** *Sedative, analgesic, anesthetic* **Uses:** *Induction agent for short diagnostic and surgical procedures; rapid sequence intubation in patients with status asthmaticus* **Adult dose:** *2 mg/kg IV over 1 min.* **SE:** *Elevation of BP and heart rate; increased bronchial secretions; may increase intracranial pressure; dramatic hallucinatory responses* **Notes:** *Recommended by some as the IV anesthetic of choice for patients with life-threatening asthma. Stimulates copious bronchial secretions. Onset of action within 30–60 sec. Rapid administration may result in hypotension and respiratory depression or apnea.*

Labetalol (Normodyne, Trandate)	**Action:** Alpha- and beta-blocker
	Uses: Hypertension
	Adult dose: 10 mg IV over 1–2 min. May be repeated at 10-minute intervals as needed to a maximum of 150 mg. Alternately, initial dose can be given IV, then IV infusion given at 2–8 mg/min.
	SE: Bradycardia, dizziness, fatigue, nausea, dyspnea
	Notes: Concurrent use with calcium channel blockers can cause severe hypotension. Do not use in asthma, COPD, heart block, uncompensated CHF, or cardiogenic shock.
Lidocaine 2% (Xylocaine)	**Action:** Class IB antiarrhythmic
	Uses: Pulseless VT/VF (if amiodarone unavailable), stable monomorphic or polymorphic VT; *pre-intubation for head trauma or intracranial bleeding; reduce bronchospasm induced by laryngoscopy and intubation*
	Adult dose:
	• VF/VT cardiac arrest: 1.0–1.5 mg/kg IVP. May give additional 0.5–0.75 mg/kg IVP every 5–10 min. for refractory VF. Maximum total dose 3 mg/kg. ET dose is 2–4 mg/kg.
	• VT with pulse, wide-complex tachycardia: Doses range from 0.5–0.75 mg/kg to 1.0–1.5 mg/kg IV (each 50 mg or less may be given over 1 min.). Repeat 0.50–0.75 mg/kg IV every 5–10 min. Maximum total dose 3 mg/kg.
	• Maintenance infusion: 1–4 mg/min.
	• *Premedication before intubation 1–2 mg/kg IVP over 30–60 sec.*
	SE: Seizures, slurred speech, altered mental status, arrythmias, hypotension
	Notes: Infusion may be mixed in D5W, D10W, or NS. Discontinue immediately if signs of toxicity observed. May cause seizures if given too quickly in patient with a pulse. *When performing RSI, administer lidocaine before opioids, sedatives, or paralytics.*
Lorazepam (Ativan)	**Action:** Benzodiazepine, sedative, anticonvulsant
	Uses: Tachycardia, hypertensive emergencies, and acute coronary syndromes caused by sympathomimetic drug toxicity (e.g. cocaine, amphetamines, others); seizures (status epilepticus)
	Adult dose:
	• Cardiac effects of drug toxicity: 2 mg IV over 2–5 min.
	• Status epilepticus: 4 mg IV over 2–5 min. (may repeat in 10–15 min.) to a total dose of 8 mg
	SE: Drowsiness, confusion, hypotension, respiratory depression
	Notes: Dilute with equal volume of NS or D5W prior to administration. May need to decrease the dose in the elderly.

(continued)

Magnesium sulfate	**Action:** Electrolyte **Uses:** Cardiac arrest if torsades de pointes or suspected hypomagnesemia is present; torsades de pointes with a pulse in the presence of hypomagnesemia; life-threatening ventricular arrhythmias related to digitalis toxicity. **Adult dose:** ● Cardiac arrest: 1–2 g diluted in 10 mL D5W IV/IO over 5–20 min. ● Torsades with pulse or AMI with hypomagnesemia: 1–2 g IV mixed in 50–100 mL D5W infuse IV over 5–60 min.; may follow with IV infusion of 0.5–1.0 g/hr to control torsades. **SE:** Hypotension with rapid administration, asystole, cardiac arrest, CNS depression, respiratory depression, muscle weakness, diminished reflexes, flushing **Notes:** Do not use if renal failure or heart block is present.
Methylprednisolone sodium succinate (Solu-Medrol)	**Action:** *Corticosteroid* **Uses:** *Anaphylaxis, allergic reactions, asthma* **Adult dose:** *Usual dose 125 mg IV over 2–3 min. (range is 40–250 mg)* **SE:** *Sodium retention, fluid retention, potassium loss, hypokalemic alkalosis, hypertension, vertigo, headache* **Notes:** *Effects may not be apparent for 4–6 hours after administration.*
Metoprolol (Lopressor)	**Action:** Beta-blocker **Uses:** ST-segment-elevation MI, non-ST-segment-elevation MI, unstable angina **Adult dose:** 5 mg IV over 5 min.; may repeat twice to a total of 15 mg over 15 min. **SE:** Bradycardia, dizziness, fatigue, nausea, dyspnea, bronchospasm, insomnia **Notes:** Concurrent use with calcium channel blockers can cause severe hypotension.
Midazolam (Versed)	**Action:** Benzodiazepine, sedative-hypnotic **Uses:** Sedation **Adult dose:** ● Sedation: 1.0–2.5 mg IV over 2 min. ● *Induction sedation for RSI: 0.07–0.3 mg/kg IVP* **SE:** Respiratory depression, respiratory arrest, hypotension, nausea, vomiting **Notes:** 3 to 4 times as potent per mg as diazepam; onset: IV 1–5 min.; monitor patient respiratory status continuously after administration.

Milrinone (Primacor)	**Action:** *Inotropic, vasodilator; phosphodiesterase inhibitor* **Uses:** *Short-term treatment of CHF, usually in patients receiving digoxin and diuretics* **Adult dose:** • *Loading dose: 50 mcg/kg IV over 10 min.* • *Maintenance (standard dose): Infuse IV at a rate of 0.375–0.75 mcg/kg/min* **SE:** *Supraventricular and ventricular arrhythmias; nausea, vomiting, hypotension* **Notes:** *Adjust infusion according to hemodynamic and clinical response. Reduce dose if renal failure is present.*
Morphine sulfate (Duramorph)	**Action:** Analgesic **Uses:** Analgesia, chest pain unresponsive to nitrates in ACS, pulmonary edema **Adult dose:** 2–4 mg IV over 1–5 min.; may repeat at 2–8 mg every 5–15 min. **SE:** Hypotension, respiratory depression, nausea, vomiting **Notes:** Reverse with naloxone if needed. Use cautiously in RV infarction.
Naloxone (Narcan)	**Action:** *Antidote; narcotic antagonist* **Uses:** *Narcotic overdose* **Adult dose:** *0.4–2.0 mg IV/IO (each 0.4 mg over 15 sec). Repeat every 2 min. if needed, up to 10 mg total dose. May give 0.4–0.8 mg IM or SC.* **SE:** *May cause narcotic withdrawal; patients with cardiovascular disease may experience arrhythmias or severe alterations in blood pressure.* **Notes:** *Effects of naloxone may not outlast narcotic effects. Give small doses slowly if known narcotic dependence. Ventilate before administration.*
Nitroglycerin (tablets— Nitrostat; spray— Nitrolingual; IV—Tridil)	**Action:** Antianginal, vasodilator **Uses:** Acute coronary syndromes, CHF, acute pulmonary edema **Adult dose:** • SL tablets: 0.3–0.4 mg; may repeat in 5 min.; maximum 3 doses • Spray: 0.4 mg (1 spray); spray under tongue at 5-minute intervals; maximum 3 doses • IV infusion: Start at 10–20 mcg/min and increase dose 5 mcg/min every 5–10 min. to desired effect. **SE:** Hypotension, headache, flushing, palpitations, syncope

(continued)

Notes: Do not administer if SBP < 90 (or > 30 mmHg below baseline SBP); do not administer if HR < 50 bpm or > 100 bpm, if RV infarct, or if drugs for erectile dysfunction used within 24 hours (sildenafil and vardenafil) or tadalafil used within 48 hours. Do not mix with other drugs in infusion.

Norepinephrine (Levophed)	**Action:** *Vasoconstrictor* **Uses:** *Severe cardiogenic shock, hemodynamically significant hypotension (systolic BP < 70 mm Hg) unresponsive to other agents* **Adult dose:** *0.5–1.0 mcg/min IV titrated to improve BP (up to 30 mcg/min)* **SE:** *May worsen myocardial ischemia, arrhythmias; infiltration will cause tissue necrosis* **Notes:** *Onset immediate; administer by IV infusion; taper off gradually. Do not give alkaline solutions in the same IV line. Do not use to treat hypovolemic shock.*

Oxygen	**Action:** Improves tissue oxygenation
	Uses: Any suspected cardiopulmonary emergency, especially complaints of shortness of breath and/or suspected ischemic chest pain; cardiopulmonary arrest
	Adult dose:
	  • Nasal cannula: 1–6 L/min, 24–44% oxygen
	  • Partial rebreather mask: 6–10 L/min, 35–60% oxygen
	  • Nonrebreather mask: 10–15 L/min, 60–100% oxygen
	  • Bag/mask: 15 L/min, up to 100% oxygen
	SE: Possible toxicity with prolonged administration of high-flow oxygen
	Notes: Pulse oximetry is inaccurate in low cardiac output states or with vasoconstriction or carbon monoxide exposure.

Physostigmine (Antilirium)	**Action:** *Antidote; short-acting cholinergic agent; reversible cholinesterase inhibitor* **Uses:** *Hemodynamically significant tachycardia associated with pure anticholinergic poisoning and tricyclic antidepressant toxicity* **Adult dose:** *0.5–2.0 mg IV over 2 min.; may repeat every 20–30 min. as needed* **SE:** *Seizures, worsened AV conduction, bradycardia, hypotension, cardiac arrest, lacrimation, salivation* **Notes:** *Very narrow therapeutic-to-toxic ratio. Do not use in the presence of GI/GU obstruction.*

Potassium chloride	**Action:** *Electrolyte replacement* **Uses:** *Hypokalemia* **Adult dose:** *10–20 mEq/hr IV; mix 40 mEq of potassium in 1 L of normal saline* **SE:** *Burning at IV site, hyperkalemia, nausea, vomiting, flatulence, abdominal pain/discomfort, diarrhea, arrhythmias* **Notes:** *Monitor ECG continuously or with serial ECGs during potassium replacement therapy. Monitor serum potassium levels to avoid undertreatment or over-treatment. Administer by central line if possible.*
Procainamide (Pronestyl)	**Action:** Class IA antiarrhythmic **Uses:** Narrow-complex SVT after vagal maneuvers and adenosine, atrial fibrillation with rapid ventricular rate in patients with WPW, stable wide-complex tachycardia of uncertain type, stable VT with normal QT interval **Adult dose:** 20 mg/min IV infusion until arrhythmia resolves, hypotension develops, QRS widens by > 50%, or total dose of 17 mg/kg is given. (In urgent situations, up to 50 mg/min may be given to total dose of 17 mg/kg). Maintenance infusion 1–4 mg/min (diluted in NS or D5W). **SE:** Hypotension, AV block, prolongation of PR, QRS, QT intervals, GI upset **Notes:** Use with caution with other drugs that prolong QT interval (e.g., amiodarone). If cardiac or renal dysfunction present, reduce maximum total dose to 12 mg/kg and maintenance infusion to 1–2 mg/min.
Propofol (Diprivan)	**Action:** Sedative, analgesic, dissociative anesthetic **Uses:** Induction agent for rapid sequence intubation; maintenance of sedation during mechanical ventilation **Adult dose:** 2.0–2.5 mg/kg IV (about 40 mg every 10 sec until onset of desired sedation); then 0.1–0.2 mg/kg/min **SE:** Anaphylaxis, angioedema, apnea, arrhythmia exacerbation, bradycardia, dystonic reaction, flushing, hyperkalemia, hypertension, hypotension, involuntary muscle movements, laryngospasm, nausea, seizures, vomiting, burning at IV site **Notes:** Possesses bronchodilator properties. Severe hypotension, respiratory depression and muscle movements possible if administered too quickly.

(continued)

Propranolol (Inderal)	**Action:** Beta-blocker; non-selective beta-adrenergic antagonist
	Uses: ST-segment-elevation MI, non-ST-segment-elevation MI, unstable angina
	Adult dose: Total dose is 0.1 mg/kg slow IV, divided into 3 equal doses at 2- to 3-minute intervals. Do not exceed 1 mg/min. Repeat after 2 min. if necessary.
	SE: Bradycardia, dizziness, fatigue, nausea, dyspnea
	Notes: Concurrent use with calcium channel blockers can cause severe hypotension. Do not use in asthma, uncompensated CHF, bradycardia, or heart block.
Reteplase, recombinant (Retavase)	**Action:** Fibrinolytic; converts plasminogen to plasmin, promoting fibrinolysis
	Uses: ST-segment-elevation MI
	Adult dose: 10 units IV over 2 min. Repeat dose in 30 min. Flush with normal saline before and after each bolus.
	SE: Bleeding, arrhythmias, hypotension, allergic reaction
	Notes: Heparin and reteplase are incompatible in solution and should not be administered via the same IV line. Heparin and aspirin should be given concurrently. Carefully screen for contraindications.
Rocuronium (Zemuron)	**Action:** *Paralytic; non-depolarizing neuromuscular blocking agent competes with acetylcholine at the nicotinic receptor site.*
	Uses: *Paralysis in rapid sequence intubation*
	Adult dose: *0.6–1.2 mg/kg IVP*
	SE: *Apnea, malignant hyperthermia, wheezing, hypertension, hypotension*
	Notes: *Onset of action is comparable to succinylcholine, but its duration of action is significantly longer. Reduce dose in hepatic impairment. Aminoglycosides, vancomycin, and tetracycline enhance blockade.*
Sodium bicarbonate	**Action:** Alkalinizing agent
	Uses: Hyperkalemia; acidosis associated with tricyclic antidepressant overdose (OD), barbiturate OD, salicylate OD, cocaine OD, diphenhydramine OD; prolonged arrest with effective ventilation; after ROSC from prolonged cardiac arrest
	Adult dose: 1 mEq/kg IVP. Continuous infusion may be mixed by adding 3 ampules of sodium bicarbonate (150 mEq) to 850 mL of D5W. Some experts recommend adding 30 mEq of potassium chloride to the IV infusion administered over 4–8 hours. Repeat IV boluses and the rate of the continuous infusion should be guided by arterial pH.

	SE: Metabolic alkalosis, fluid overload, hypernatremia **Notes:** Extravasation may manifest ulceration, sloughing, cellulitis, or tissue necrosis at the IV site. Incompatible with many ACLS drugs; flush IV tubing with NS before and after administration.
Sodium nitroprusside (Nipride)	**Action:** *Arterial and venous vasodilator* **Uses:** *Hypertensive crisis* **Adult dose:** *Begin IV infusion at 0.1 mcg/kg/min and titrate upward every 3–5 min. to desired effect (up to 5 mcg/kg/min)* **SE:** *Hypotension, thiocyanate toxicity, palpitations, headache, GI upset* **Notes:** *Use with an infusion pump; wrap in foil or other opaque material*
Sodium polystyrene sulfonate (Kayexalate)	**Actions:** *Cation-exchange resin that binds potassium and eliminates it from the GI tract* **Uses:** *Hyperkalemia* **Adult dose:** *15–60 g PO or 30–60 grams PR every 6 hours based on serum potassium* **SE:** *Anorexia, constipation, GI obstruction, hypokalemia, hypocalcemia, muscle weakness, nausea/vomiting, sodium retention* **Notes:** *Dosage must be individualized; monitor total body potassium. Use with caution if CHF, edema, and/or hypertension is present. Takes hours to days to correct hyperkalemia; use other measures to correct severe hyperkalemia rapidly.*
Streptokinase (Streptase)	**Action:** Fibrinolytic; converts plasminogen to plasmin, promoting fibrinolysis **Uses:** ST-segment-elevation MI **Adult dose:** 1.5 million IU infused IV over 60 min. **SE:** Chest pain or arrhythmias due to reperfusion, bleeding, hypotension, allergic reaction, bronchospasm, internal bleeding **Notes:** Increased risk of bleeding in elderly patients. Do not use if streptococcal infection or streptokinase use in last 6 months. Carefully screen for contraindications.
Succinylcholine (Anectine)	**Action:** *Paralytic; depolarizing neuromuscular blocking agent* **Uses:** *Paralysis in rapid sequence intubation* **Adult dose:** *1–2 mg/kg IVP* **SE:** *Apnea, malignant hyperthermia, arrhythmias, muscle fasciculations, rise in intracranial pressure, hyperkalemia, hypertension* **Notes:** *Onset 1–2 min. Paralyzed patients must also be given sedatives. Do not use if renal failure, burns, hyperkalemia*

(continued)

Tenecteplase (TNKase)	**Action:** Fibrinolytic; converts plasminogen to plasmin, promoting fibrinolysis **Uses:** ST-segment-elevation MI **Adult dose:** 30–50 mg IVP over 5 seconds, based on patient weight: • < 60 kg: 30 mg • 60–69 kg: 35 mg • 70–79 kg: 40 mg • 80–89 kg: 45 mg • 90+ kg: 50 mg **SE:** Bleeding, allergic reaction, arrhythmias **Notes:** Incompatible with dextrose solutions. Flush line with NS before and after administration. Carefully screen for contraindications.
Vasopressin (Pitressin)	**Action:** Potent vasoconstrictor **Uses:** May replace first or second epinephrine dose in cardiac arrest **Adult dose:** 40 units, IVP/IO **SE:** Wheezing, hives, hypertension, arrhythmias, vertigo **Notes:** Not recommended for responsive patients with coronary artery disease; may be useful in vasodilatory shock (e.g., septic shock).
Vecuronium (Norcuron)	**Action:** *Paralytic; nondepolarizing neuromuscular blocker that competes with acetylcholine at the nicotinic receptor site* **Uses:** *Paralysis in rapid sequence intubation* **Adult dose:** *0.1–0.2 mg/kg IVP* **SE:** *Apnea, minimal cardiovascular side effects, tachycardia, bradycardia* **Notes:** *Onset 1–2 min. Paralyzed patients must also be given sedatives.*
Verapamil (Isoptin, Calan)	**Action:** Calcium channel blocker; slows AV node conduction, slows HR, decreases force of contraction, peripheral vasodilation, reduces myocardial oxygen consumption **Uses:** Narrow-QRS PSVT; atrial fibrillation, flutter, or multifocal atrial tachycardia with rapid ventricular response **Adult dose:** 2.5–5.0 mg IV over 2–3 min. May repeat with 5–10 mg IV over 2–3 min. every 15–30 min. up to 20 mg. (Alternative dose: 5 mg IV over 2–3 min. every 15 min. up to 30 mg.) **SE:** Hypotension, AV block, bradycardia, asystole **Notes:** Avoid in WPW and wide-QRS tachycardia and cardiogenic shock.

Sources:
- American Heart Association (2005). "Guidelines for CPR and ECC." *Circulation* 112:IV.
- American Heart Association (2006). *Handbook of Emergency Cardiovascular Care*. Dallas, Tx.
- David J. Roberts (2002). "Common Cardiovascular Drugs." Chap. 146 in *Rosen's Emergency Medicine: Concepts and Clinical Practice*, 5th ed. Ed.-in-chief J. A. Marx. Mosby.
- Gahart, B., and A. Nazareno. (2005). *Intravenous Medications*. Mosby.
- Mosby Elsevier (2006). *Mosby's Drug Consult for Health Professions*. Mosby.

Common ACLS Abbreviations

ABCD	airway–breathing–circulation–defibrillation
ABG	arterial blood gas
ACE	angiotensin-converting enzyme
ACLS	advanced cardiac life support
ACS	acute coronary syndrome
AED	automated external defibrillator
a-fib	atrial fibrillation
AF	atrial flutter
AHA	American Heart Association
AICD	automatic implantable cardioverter/defibrillator
AMI	acute myocardial infarction
aPTT	activated partial thromboplastin time
ASA	aspirin
AV	atrioventricular
AVM	arteriovenous malformation
BiPAP	bi-level positive airway pressure
BLS	basic life support
BP	blood pressure
BPM	beats per minute
BVM	bag-valve-mask
BVT	bag-valve-tube
CABG	coronary artery bypass graft
CAD	coronary artery disease
CBC	complete blood count
CHF	congestive heart failure

CK-MB	creatine kinase–myocardial bands
CO_2	carbon dioxide
COPD	chronic obstructive pulmonary disease
CPAP	continuous positive airway pressure
CPR	cardiopulmonary resuscitation
CT	computed tomography
CVA	cerebrovascular accident
CXR	chest X-ray
D5W	5% dextrose in water
DBP	diastolic blood pressure
defib	defibrillation
DNAR	do not attempt resuscitation
DNR	do not resuscitate
DVT	deep vein thrombosis
ECC	emergency cardiovascular care
ECG	electrocardiogram
ED	emergency department
EDD	esophageal detection device
EF	ejection fraction
EMS	emergency medical services
ET	endotracheal
ETC	esophageal-tracheal Combitube
$ETCO_2$	end-tidal carbon dioxide
ETT	endotracheal tube
FBAO	foreign body airway obstruction
FRC	functional residual capacity

g	gram
GP	glycoprotein
Hg	mercury
HR	heart rate
Hx	history
ICH	intracranial hemorrhage
INR	international normalized ratio
IO	intraosseous
ITD	impedance threshold device
IV	intravenous
IVP	intravenous push
kg	kilogram
LAD	left anterior descending (coronary artery)
LAPSS	Los Angeles Prehospital Stroke Screen
LBBB	left bundle branch block
LCX	left coronary artery, circumflex branch
LMA	laryngeal mask airway
L/min	liters per minute
LMWH	low-molecular-weight heparin
LPM	liters per minute
LR	lactated ringers solution
LV	left ventricular
MAT	multifocal atrial tachycardia
mcg	micrograms
mg	milligrams
MI	myocardial infarction
min	minutes
mm	millimeters
NPA	nasopharyngeal airway
NS	normal saline (0.9%NaCL)
NSAID	nonsteroidal anti-inflammatory drug
NSR	normal sinus rhythm
NSTEMI	non-ST-segment-elevation myocardial infarction
NTG	nitroglycerin
O$_2$	oxygen
ODS	osmotic demyelination syndrome
OPA	oropharyngeal airway

PAT	paroxysmal atrial tachycardia
PCI	percutaneous coronary intervention
PE	pulmonary embolism
PEA	pulseless electrical activity
PEEP	positive end-expiratory pressure
PEF	peak expiratory flow
PIH	pregnancy-induced hypertension
PSVT	paroxysmal supraventricular tachycardia
PT	prothrombin time
PVCs	premature ventricular contractions
RCA	right coronary artery
RSI	rapid sequence intubation
RV	right ventricular
SAH	subarachnoid hemorrhage
SBP	systolic blood pressure
SC	subcutaneous
sec	seconds
SIADH	syndrome of inappropriate antidiuretic hormone secretion
SL	sublingual
STEMI	ST-segment-elevation myocardial infarction
SVR	systemic vascular resistance
SVT	supraventricular tachycardia
TCA	tricyclic antidepressant
TCP	transcutaneous pacing
TdP	torsades de pointes
TIA	transient ischemic attack
TIMI	thrombolysis in myocardial infarction
TKO	to keep open
tPA	tissue plasminogen activator
UA	unstable angina
UFH	unfractionated heparin
VF	ventricular fibrillation
VT	ventricular tachycardia
WPW	Wolff-Parkinson-White (syndrome)

Index

PARENT HEART WATCH

Parent Heart Watch (PHW) is a state-by-state network of parents and partners dedicated to reducing the often disastrous effects of sudden cardiac arrest (SCA) in children. Parent Heart Watch was established by parents for parents and families that have been affected by SCA throughout the United States. The parents involved with Parent Heart Watch have worked with legislators on the state and federal level to pass laws that require automated external defibrillators (AEDs) in schools, on athletic playing fields, and in fitness centers, public buildings, senior centers, golf courses, and stadiums. It is our goal to see AEDs in every public place so that communities are more comfortable using them when they are needed.

Through this state-by-state network, these families have been empowering each other to turn their tragedy into positive efforts for families and communities across the nation. Parent Heart Watch enables information sharing, support networks, and the formulation of nationwide programs that meet our mission and objectives.

In addition to helping in the fight against SCA, Parent Heart Watch is a support system for those who have already been affected by the loss of a beloved child that is so unexpected. Children who die of SCA are most often free of symptoms that would alert anyone to a preexisting cardiac condition. These children usually pass school and athletic physicals with flying colors.

In 2006, Parent Heart Watch held its inaugural leadership forum for families who have lost children to SCA. This forum was designed so that families could attend seminars to help them cope with loss and also to learn to comfort one another through the creation of programs that educate the public about SCA.

During the 2006 forum, members were provided with facts and information to help drive change in their communities. Information-sharing seminars were held by cardiologists, AED manufacturers, and parents who had already made a visible effort in their communities. Their efforts have brought education and awareness about SCA to the forefront, sparking a collaborative effort to mandate a change in attitudes toward SCA.

This forum transformed Parent Heart Watch from a group of grieving families to a strong working foundation. These families from across the nation are now working toward change by sharing their knowledge and helping save lives, one beat at a time.

Parent Heart Watch will hold an annual forum to continue delivering tools, resources, and coaching to empower parents and members interested in carrying out the true mission of the foundation: advocating for awareness and change in the fight against SCA.

For additional information, membership forms, and parent speakers, please contact Rachel Moyer at 570-620-8338 or Rachel@parentheartwatch.org.

Rachel Moyer, Board President
Director of AED Placement and Advocacy Programs
Parent Heart Watch